Mustafa Karahan
Gino M.M.J. Kerkhoffs
Pietro Randelli • Gabriëlle J.M. Tuijthof
Editors

Effective Training of Arthroscopic Skills

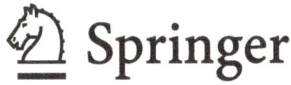
Springer

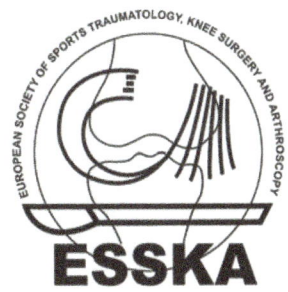
ESSKA

Editors

Mustafa Karahan
Dept. of Orthopedics and Traumatology
Acibadem University
School of Medicine
Istanbul, Turkey

Pietro Randelli
Policlinico San Donato
San Donato Milanese,
Milano, Italy

ESSKA ASBL
Centre Médical
Fondation Norbert Metz
76, rue d'Eich
1460 Luxembourg
Luxembourg

Gino M.M.J. Kerkhoffs
Department of Orthopedic Surgery
Academic Medical Centre Amsterdam
University of Amsterdam
Amsterdam, The Netherlands

Gabriëlle J.M. Tuijthof
BioMechanical Engineering
Delft University of Technology
Delft, The Netherlands

ISBN 978-3-662-44942-4   ISBN 978-3-662-44943-1   (eBook)
DOI 10.1007/978-3-662-44943-1
Springer Heidelberg New York Dordrecht London

Library of Congress Control Number: 2014956925

Springer is part of Springer Science+Business Media (www.springer.com)

Effective Training of Arthroscopic Skills

Preface

We are gratified to offer you this ESSKA Education book that represents the state-of-the-art knowledge, methods, and tools for effectively training arthroscopic skills. The European Society of Sports Traumatology, Knee Surgery and Arthroscopy (ESSKA) is highly active in promoting education of arthroscopy and arthroscopic skills in many different settings, e.g., the biannual congress, fellowship programs, and accredited teaching centers.

With the start of the ESSKA Basic Arthroscopy Course (EBAC) in Istanbul in November 2013 and the birth of the ESSKA Academy, it was time to provide all members, educators, residents, and enthusiasts for arthroscopy and arthroscopic skills training with a comprehensible overview of the state-of-the-art knowledge, methods, tools, and developments on the training of arthroscopic skills. The book covers the entire range of disciplines that contribute to an effective training of arthroscopy; it brings together themes and professionals and facilitates learning from each other to design successful and effective training programs. Above all, we hope that the book is so practical that it inspires you to embrace new technologies and methods and to start implementing them straightaway in a well-thought, evidence-based manner.

We acknowledge the great efforts of the authors, who are all experts in their field, that allowed us to present this book. Even though it is through the old-fashioned way of reading, we hope you will enjoy reading the book, perhaps with an innovative touch to it when reading on a digital e-reader!

Istanbul, Turkey   Mustafa Karahan
Amsterdam, The Netherlands   Gino M.M.J. Kerkhoffs
Milan, Italy   Pietro S. Randelli
Delft, Amsterdam, The Netherlands   Gabriëlle J.M. Tuijthof

Contents

Contributors

Umut Akgün Department of Orthopedics and Traumatology, Acibadem University School of Medicine, Istanbul, Turkey

Kash Akhtar Trauma & Orthopaedic Surgery, Imperial College Healthcare NHS Trust, London, UK

Abtin Alvand, BSc(Hons), MBBS, MRCS(Eng) Nuffield Department of Orthopaedic Surgery, Nuffield Orthopaedic Centre, Oxford, UK

Federico Cabitza Dipartimento di Informatica Sistemistica e Comunicazione, Universita' degli Studi di Milano-Bicocca, Milan, Italy

Riccardo Compagnoni, MD Dipartimento Di Scienze Medico-Chirurgiche, Università Degli Studi Di Milano, IRCCS, Policlinico San Donato, Milan, Italy

Jenny Dankelman Department of Biomechanical Engineering, Delft University of Technology, Delft, The Netherlands

Dutch Arthrocopy Society Teaching committee (DAST) Nederlandse Vereniging voor Arthroscopie, Tilburg, The Netherlands

Jamie Y. Ferguson Nuffield Department of Orthopaedics, Rheumatology and Musculoskeletal Sciences, University of Oxford, Oxford, UK

Chinmay M. Gupte, MRCS Biomechanics Section, Departments of Bioengineering and Mechanical Engineering, Imperial College London, London, UK

Tim Horeman Department of Biomechanical Engineering, Delft University of Technology, Delft, The Netherlands

Mustafa Karahan Department of Orthopedics and Traumatology, Acibadem University School of Medicine, Istanbul, Turkey

Gino M.M.J. Kerkhoffs Department of Orthopedic Surgery, Academic Medical Centre, Amsterdam, The Netherlands

Izaäk F. Kodde Department of Orthopedic Surgery, Academic Medical Centre, Amsterdam, The Netherlands

Jan Maarten Luursema Department of Surgery, UMC Radboud, Nijmegen, The Netherlands

Hermann O. Mayr, MD Department of Orthopedic and Trauma Surgery, Albert Ludwig University of Freiburg, Freiburg, Germany

Andrew J. Price, MD Nuffield Department of Orthopaedic Surgery, Nuffield Orthopaedic Centre, Oxford, UK

Vincenza Ragone, MSc Me Dipartimento Di Scienze Medico-Chirurgiche, Università Degli Studi Di Milano, IRCCS, Policlinico San Donato, Milan, Italy

Pietro S. Randelli, MD Dipartimento di Scienze Biomediche per la Salute, Università degli Studi di Milano, Milan, Italy

Jonathan L. Rees, MD Nuffield Department of Orthopaedics, Rheumatology and Musculoskeletal Sciences, University of Oxford, Oxford, UK

Kevin Sherman, MD Department of Orthopedics, Castle Hill Hospital, Cottingham, East Yorkshire, UK

Inger N. Sierevelt, MSc Department of Orthopedics, Slotervaart Hospital, Amsterdam, The Netherlands

Nigel J. Standfield Trauma & Orthopaedic Surgery, Imperial College Healthcare NHS Trust, London, UK

Amelie Stöhr Department of Orthopedic and Trauma Surgery, Albert Ludwig University of Freiburg, Freiburg, Germany

Gabriëlle J.M. Tuijthof Department of Biomechanical Engineering, Delft University of Technology, Delft, The Netherlands

Department of Orthopedic SurgeryAcademic Medical Centre, Amsterdam, The Netherlands

John J. van den Dobbelsteen Department of Biomechanical Engineering, Delft University of Technology, Delft, The Netherlands

Obstacles Faced in the Classical Training System: Why Is There a Need for Newer Systems?

1

Pietro S. Randelli, Mustafa Karahan, Jamie Y. Ferguson, Kash Akhtar, and Kevin Sherman

Take-Home Message
Times have changed, some may have the gift to become an excellent surgeon, but it is possible to raise a surgeon with proper training.

1.1 Introduction and Statements

A surgeon's anatomy is multifaceted. To be an experienced surgeon, one requires a depth of cognitive knowledge, an appropriate surgical judgment, and an ability to act quickly but thoughtfully and, when necessary, in a decisive manner (Wanzel et al. 2002). The surgeon must be dedicated and perceptive, have spontaneous compassion, and be a good communicator. Surgeons should be excellent in surgical craftsmanship to perform particular technical tasks. A contemporary concept of surgical education requires all to be included in a program from the standpoint of educational objectives, educational curricula, and assessment mechanisms.

Surgical residency programs have a history of almost 100 years and the structure has not changed appreciably (Bell 2004). William S. Halsted established a graduate training program for surgeons based on the German System at the Johns Hopkins Hospital. When the American Board of Surgery was organized in 1937, the Halsted triad of educational principles was the goal of the founders: knowledge of the basic sciences, research, and graduated patient responsibility for the resident (Sealy 1999). Halsted's system was a pyramidal structure characterized by indefinite length, vigorous competition for advancement leaving only one resident at the pinnacle and one chief of service.

Traditional surgical training based on Halsted's program was described as cruel to patients and inexcusably demanding of residents with little emphasis on education (Pories 1999). The system resulted in success only when the resident was bright, devoted to care, and technically capable and failed when

P.S. Randelli, MD (✉)
Aggregato in Ortopedia e Traumatologia,
Dipartimento di Scienze Biomediche per la Salute,
Università degli Studi di Milano,
IRCCS Policlinico San Donato, Milan, Italy
e-mail: pietro.randelli@unimi.it

M. Karahan
Department of Orthopedics and Traumatology,
Acibadem University School of Medicine,
Istanbul, Turkey
e-mail: drmustafakarahan@gmail.com

J.Y. Ferguson
Nuffield Department of Orthopaedics,
Rheumatology and Musculoskeletal Sciences,
University of Oxford, Oxford, UK

K. Akhtar
Trauma and Orthopaedic Surgery,
Imperial College Healthcare NHS Trust, London, UK
e-mail: surgery@me.com; kasurgery@gmail.com

K. Sherman, MD
Department of Orthopedics, Castle Hill Hospital,
Cottingham, East Yorkshire, UK
e-mail: kp_sherman@hotmail.com

residents were "average" or when the problem was complex. Despite the inferior conditions for the residents, residents learned to bond, to share knowledge, and to work as a team. Many in that generation became the pioneers of surgery, immunology, molecular biology, and technology. However, in some institutions, only 20 % of the residents completed their program of their initial choice; the rest had to move to inferior programs.

Times have changed and extrinsic conditions are influencing ways in which trainees learn.

1.2   Economy-Driven Patient Care

Fast pace of innovation in surgical techniques, combined with patient safety issues, limited operating room resources, and limited resident work hours, has yielded new paradigms for surgical education (Morris et al. 1993).

1.3   Liability Issues

Surgeons as part of the medical practitioners are no longer employers. They are seen as providers to a system and no longer considered the ultimate decision makers in the flow charts of patient care. Unfortunately, decisions are based on health economics driven by the payers of the health care. As a consequence of these developments, surgery settings have moved from large hospitals to smaller outpatient surgery clinics where costs are relatively lower. However, outpatient surgical clinics are far from being an ideal surgical training setting.

As a consequence of a combination of factors such as society evolution, increase in public awareness, and soaring health-care costs, physicians' responsibility for their malpractices has increased unrelated to their income. The surgeon has financial issues at stake in addition to the responsibility inherent to the nature of the profession. This is one more reason why a surgeon should not take the responsibility of a patient before he is fully proficient.

1.4   Limited Working Hours

Health policies and workers' regulations in certain regions limit working hours. European Working Time Regulation on numbers of hours in which surgical trainees are available to be taught means that exposure to clinical materials and operating opportunities is restricted (O'Neill et al. 2002; Wirth et al. 2014).

1.5   Rapid Advances in Surgical Techniques

Surgery in the current era cannot be performed without instruments unlike the era when the classical teaching methods were set. Most of the instruments are universal and used throughout training. However, certain instruments or devices are unique to the surgery performed and the resident has to get familiar with them prior to the operating room.

1.6   Evolution of the Trainee and the Trainer

Unlike the times of Halsted's program, current residents are products of a society where demanding training is considered as a rightful claim, and trainers are expected to be more active in teaching compared to previous terms. As adult learning principles are integrated more into surgical training, individual characteristics of trainees are assessed for a better and more effective training. Recent data has shown that learners have preferences for the ways in which they receive and process information. The VARK model categorizes learners as visual (V), aural (A), read/write (R), and kinesthetic (K) (Kim et al. 2013).

1.7   Evolution of Information Technology in the Digital Era

Digital Age has influenced medical practice along with how information is transferred. Medical and surgical training is one of the areas that advances in information technology (IT) had its impact on. Out of all, residents who are the recipients of the training had their development within the Internet age. Various combinations of training are under question such as the role of medical students in the training of junior residents (Wirth et al. 2014). These folks are dynamic, lenient toward faster pace in exchange of information, and aware of the changes around. They are well informed. In addition to the recipient, means of training is more different than before, i.e., simulation through virtual reality did not exist in Halsted's times. Internet has reformed not only medicine but the whole humanity. Researches are using benefits that the modern age is offering us. In addition to the changes within our field, a lot of changes have taken place in those related to education. There are well-developed concepts in educational psychology that may be used in developing improved methods to assess and train prospective surgeons.

Conclusion

Finally, we are able to make a clear description of the fundamentals of surgical training that did not exist a century ago (Thomas 2008):

> Clearly defined selection criteria
> An efficient, fair and transparent selection process
> A "fit for purpose" learning environment
> Appropriate access for trainees to clinical practice
> Trained motivated trainers
> An integrated progression of learning
> Effective and objective assessment of competency progression

We, physicians, while following guidelines provided to us by our masters and sustaining the soul of our profession, will be able to generate successful surgeons for the future.

Bibliography

Bell RH Jr (2004) Alternative training models for surgical residency. Surg Clin North Am 84(6):1699–1711, xii available from: PM:15501282

Kim RH, Gilbert T, Ristig K, Chu QD (2013) Surgical resident learning styles: faculty and resident accuracy at identification of preferences and impact on ABSITE scores. J Surg Res 184(1):31–36, available from: PM:23706561

Morris AH, Jennings JE, Stone RG, Katz JA, Garroway RY, Hendler RC (1993) Guidelines for privileges in arthroscopic surgery. Arthroscopy 9(1):125–127, available from: PM:8442822

O'Neill PJ, Cosgarea AJ, Freedman JA, Queale WS, McFarland EG (2002) Arthroscopic proficiency: a survey of orthopaedic sports medicine fellowship directors and orthopaedic surgery department chairs. Arthroscopy 18(7):795–800, available from: PM:12209439

Pories W (1999) Some reflections on Halsted and residency training. Curr Surg 56(1–2):1

Sealy W (1999) Halsted is dead: time for change in graduate surgical education. Curr Surg 56(1–2):34–38

Thomas W (2008) The making of a surgeon. Surgery (Oxford) 26(10):400–402

Wanzel KR, Ward M, Reznick RK (2002) Teaching the surgical craft: from selection to certification. Curr Probl Surg 39(6):573–659, available from: PM:12037512

Wirth K, Malone B, Barrera K, Widmann WD, Turner C, Sanni A (2014) Is there a place for medical students as teachers in the education of junior residents? Am J Surg 207(2):271–274, available from: PM:24468027

Part I

Psychomotor Skills: Learning and Education

Needs and Wishes from the Arthroscopy Community

2

Pietro S. Randelli, Federico Cabitza,
Vincenza Ragone, Riccardo Compagnoni,
Kash Akhtar, and Gabriëlle J.M. Tuijthof
Dutch Arthroscopy Society Teaching committee (DAST)

Take-Home Messages
- Residents need to learn many skills before performing safely independent in the operating theatre.
- A quality training program should focus on skills that are considered more important for performing arthroscopy: anatomical knowledge, triangulation, and spatial perception.
- Online surveys can be useful to investigate the opinion and generate consensus from orthopedic surgeons about what should be trained and skills that are crucial for a resident to possess before continuing safe in the operating room.
- Training simulators should focus on skills considered more relevant by a large number of physicians:
  - Portal placement
  - Anatomical knowledge on identification of different compartments, intercondylar notch including ACL and PCL, and all important structures in the joint
  - Inspection with the arthroscope

2.1 Introduction

Surgical skills training plays an important role in medical education. In recent years, substantial progress has been made in the development of simulation programs and tools for the training and assessment of a trainee's performance. However, these devices have generated controversy about their validity for arthroscopic surgical training,

P.S. Randelli, MD (✉)
Dipartimento di Scienze Biomediche per la Salute,
Università degli Studi di Milano, Milan, Italy
e-mail: pietro.randelli@unimi.it

F. Cabitza
Dipartimento di Informatica Sistemistica e
Comunicazione, Universita' degli Studi di
Milano-Bicocca, Milan, Italy
e-mail: cabitza@disco.unimib.it

V. Ragone, MSc Me • R. Compagnoni, MD
Dipartimento Di Scienze Medico-Chirurgiche,
Università Degli Studi Di Milano, IRCCS,
Policlinico San Donato, Milan, Italy
e-mail: ragone.vincenza@inwind.it;
riccardo.compagnoni@gmail.com

K. Akhtar
Trauma and Orthopaedic Surgery,
Imperial College Healthcare NHS Trust, London, UK
e-mail: surgery@me.com; kasurgery@gmail.com

G.J.M. Tuijthof
Department of Biomechanical Engineering,
Delft University of Technology,
Delft, The Netherlands

Department of Orthopedic Surgery,
Academic Medical Centre,
Amsterdam, The Netherlands
e-mail: g.j.m.tuijthof@tudelft.nl

Dutch Arthroscopy Society Teaching committee (DAST)
Nederlandse Vereniging voor Arthroscopie,
Nieuwe Bosscheweg 9, Tilburg 5017 JJ,
The Netherlands
e-mail: NVA@scopie.org

and the bridge between technological development and educational needs has not yet been clearly established. From an educational point of view, a key feature for a well-designed training program is that the learning objectives should be explicitly defined (Biggs 2003). The aim of this chapter is to address the learning objectives in simulation training, and subsequently, we focus on the number of procedures that are required to become competent.

2.2 Learning Objectives for Simulation Training

Only few studies to date have tried to determine the relevance of skills that a simulator or training protocol should teach to residents. Concerning what skills are crucial for a resident to possess before continuing safe training in the operating room, results of a questionnaire submitted to the members of the Canadian association of orthopedic surgeon are available in the literature (Safir et al. 2008). The online survey outlining fundamental skills of arthroscopy and methods that a surgical trainee might use to develop such skills was composed of 35 questions. Surgeons were asked to rank the importance of each arthroscopic task or usefulness of a learning method on a five-point scale ranging from least important to most important. Overall, 101 orthopedic surgeons responded to survey. Anatomy

identification and navigation skills were deemed to be the most important for a trainee to possess prior to entering the operating room (Table 2.1). Furthermore, portal positioning and triangulation were elected as the most important specific skills.

Hui and coworkers (2013) reported results of 65 orthopedic residents that completed online a similar survey. Identification of structures and navigation of the arthroscope were ranked highly in terms of importance for trainee surgeons to possess before performing in the operating room (Table 2.1).

Supported by the Dutch Arthroscopy Society (NVA), a similar questionnaire was conducted in the Netherlands among the experienced arthroscopists and residents to determine the presence of cultural differences. The preliminary results of the Dutch survey are presented together with the results from Safir and coworkers (2008) and Hui and coworkers (2013) (Table 2.1). In all three surveys, knowledge on anatomy of the knee joint is ranked as priority number one.

In order to investigate the opinion of a large community of orthopedic surgeons, an online survey was distributed to surgeons that are members of the European Society of Sports Traumatology, Knee Surgery & Arthroscopy (ESSKA) and among the members of the Dutch Arthroscopy Society. The purpose of the project was to generate consensus from a group of experienced orthopedic surgeons about what should be trained and

Table 2.1 Ranking of importance for a trainee to possess ability prior to performing in the operating room

Rank	Surgeons (Safir et al. 2008) $n=101$	Score (1–5)	Residents (Hui et al. 2013) $n=67$	Score (1–5)	Surgeons-residents NVA $n=20$	Score (1–5)	Surgeons-residents $n=195$	Score (1–5)
1	Anatomical knowledge	3.86[a]	Anatomical knowledge	4.4	Anatomical knowledge	4.70	Anatomical knowledge	4.63[b]
2	Triangulation/depth perception	3.34[a]	Spatial perception	4.3	Spatial perception	4.15	Triangulation	4.43[b]
3	Spatial perception	2.77[a]	Triangulation/depth perception	4.2	Tactile sensation	4.15	Spatial perception	4.29[b]
4	Manual dexterity	2.86[a]	Manual dexterity	4.2	Manual dexterity	4.00	Tactile sensation	4.00[b]
5	Tactile sensation	2.05[a]	Tactile sensation	3.7	Triangulation	3.75	Manual dexterity	3.85[b]

[a]Significantly different ($p<0.001$) (Safir et al. 2008)
[b]Significantly different ($p<0.001$), this chapter

skills that are crucial for a resident to possess before continuing safe in the operating room.

An online survey was developed based upon the questions Safir and coworkers asked (Safir et al. 2008) and distributed using an open-source platform (www.limesurvey.org). An e-mail to present the research initiative and to invite to complete the online questionnaire was sent to about 1,000 members of ESSKA.

The survey on training knee arthroscopy encompassed 65 questions outlining fundamental skills of arthroscopy and methods that a surgical trainee might use to develop such skills. The survey consisted of 5 questions regarding generic skills and 10 regarding specific skills; 16 items about patient and tissue manipulation, 11 about knowledge of pathology, and 6 about inspection of the anatomical structures; 5 questions concerning practice methods to prepare residents; 3 items about global exercises; and 9 about detailed exercises that residents have to be trained for (Tables 2.2, 2.3, 2.4, 2.5, and 2.6).

Surgeons were asked to indicate the importance of each arthroscopic task on a six-point ordinal scale with explicit anchors at the extremes ranging from *not important at all* (score 1) to *very important* (score 6) in order to increase response variance while better discriminating central tendency bias. The results were later down sampled to a 5-point scale to guarantee comparability to other studies (the univariate analysis of the information lost in the down sampling would be out of the scope of the chapter) (Hui et al. 2013;

Table 2.3 Results of specific skills

Specific skills	Priority level	Rank	Median	Mean
Sterility	Level 1[a]	1	5	4.6
Knowledge of pathology	Level 1[a]	2	5	4.37
Patient positioning	Level 1[a]	3	5	4.33
Preparation before the start of the operation	Level 1[a]	4	5	4.3
Knowledge of equipment	Level 1[a]	5	4	4.2
Workup	Level 1[b]	6	4	4.09
Contact with patient	Level 1, ns	7	4	4.13
Tissue manipulation	Level 1, ns	8	4	4.05
Hand positions	Level 2, ns	9	4	3.95
Overall control in the OR	Level 2, ns	9	4	3.95

ns not significant
Level 1: high-level priority. Level 2: low-level priority
[a]Items with $p < 0.001$
[b]Items with $p < 0.05$

Safir et al. 2008). Average completion time was 10.5 min and half (mean = 10.7 min, standard deviation = 7.1 min). The survey was kept open for 21 days, from the 5th of December 2013 to the 26th of the same month.

Statistical analyses were carried out using SPSS software. Results were considered statistically significant at the confidence level of 95 %, when P values were below the 5 % threshold. In order to verify whether the proposed items were considered significantly important for a novice resident, all responses were recodified in dichotomic variables considering scores of 1 and 2 as *not important* and scores of 4 and 5 as *important*. A chi-square test was conducted on the equality of response proportions *important* vs. *not important*. The 3 s in the middle were not included in this analysis for the down sampling process mentioned above; however, since those responses represented the opinion of the uncertain respondents, the verification of any polarization in the response distribution was not undermined by this discard. The rejection of the null hypothesis of

Table 2.2 Results of general skills

General skills	Priority level	Rank	Median	Mean
Anatomical knowledge	Level 1[a]	1	5	4.63
Triangulation	Level 1[a]	2	5	4.43
Spatial perception	Level 1[a]	3	4	4.29
Tissue manipulation	Level 1[a]	4	4	4
Manual dexterity	Level 1[a]	5	4	3.85

Level 1: high-level priority
[a]Items with $p < 0.001$

Table 2.4 Detailed results on patient and tissue manipulation, knowledge and pathology, and inspection of anatomical structures

Patient and tissue manipulation	Priority level	Rank	Median	Mean
Precise portal placement	Level 1[a]	1	5	4.56
Triangulating the tip of the probe with a 30° scope	Level 1[a]	2	5	4.41
Insertion of the arthroscope	Level 1[a]	3	4	4.23
Patient positioning	Level 1[a]	4	4	4.29
Entry of all compartments (medial/lateral/posteromedial, suprapatellar/intercondylar)	Level 1[a]	5	4	4.24
Judgment ligament stability (VKB, AKB, MCB, LCB)	Level 1[b]	6	4	3.74
Removal of loose bodies with grasping forceps	Level 1, ns	7	4	4.02
Joint stressing and holding of the leg	Level 2, ns	8	4	4.03
Palpation of articular surfaces with probe	Level 2, ns	9	4	3.98
How to find insertion needle	Level 2, ns	10	4	3.95
Shaving of synovium, cartilage, and meniscus	Level 2, ns	11	4	3.88
Placement of tourniquet	Level 2[b]	12	4	3.77
Exiting the joint and site closure	Level 2[a]	13	4	4.14
Use of vaporisator	Level 2[a]	14	3	3.21
Triangulating the tip of the probe with a 70° scope	Level 2[a]	15	3	3.1
Triangulating the tip of the probe with a 0° scope	Level 2[a]	16	3	2.95
Knowledge				
Knowledge of knee anatomy	Level 1[a]	1	5	4.73
Knowledge of sterility	Level 1[a]	2	5	4.48
Knowledge of ACL/PCL ruptures	Level 1[a]	3	4	4.26
Knowledge of sequence of inspection round in the knee	Level 1[a]	4	5	4.34
Knowledge of different types of meniscal tears	Level 1[a]	5	4	4.25
Knowledge of chondropathy (Outerbridge classification)	Level 1[a]	6	4	4.09
Knowledge of osteochondral defects	Level 1, ns	7	4	4.04
Knowledge of arthroscopy tower and instruments	Level 1, ns	8	4	4.04
Knowledge of corpus liberum	Level 2, ns	9	4	3.81
Knowledge of plica synovialis	Level 2[c]	10	4	3.79
Knowledge of Hoffa impingement	Level 2[a]	11	4	3.56
Navigation				
Inspection/identification of medial compartment: MFC, MTP, MM	Level 1[a]	1	5	4.4
Inspection/identification of intercondylar notch, including ACL and PCL	Level 1[a]	2	5	4.41
Inspection/identification of lateral compartment: LFC, LTP, LM	Level 1[a]	3	5	4.41
Inspection/identification of suprapatellar pouch and patellofemoral joint	Level 1[a]	4	4	4.27
Inspection/identification of lateral gutter	Level 1[a]	5	4	4.16
Inspection/identification of medial gutter	Level 1[a]	6	4	4.12

ns not significant

Level 1: high-level priority. Level 2: low-level priority

[a]Items with $p < 0.001$

[b]Items with $p < 0.05$

[c]Items with $p < 0.01$

equal proportions means that the respondents significantly assigned a high (or low) importance to the proposed items.

A qualitative ranking method was developed to identify the top-ranked items for a trainee to possess before entering an operating room. We performed the ranking of the features not by calculating the arithmetic mean of the single evaluations collected for each feature, which is a sort of conventional method for similar purposes. Indeed, this operation would be of little interest for ordinal values because

Table 2.5 Simulator preference

Simulator	Priority level	Rank	Median	Mean
Cadaveric specimen	Level 1[a]	1	5	4.27
Virtual reality simulator	Level 1[a]	2	4	3.67
Physical knee phantom equipped with sensors to track performance	Level 1[a]	3	3	3.56
Physical knee phantom (e.g., Sawbones model)	Level 1[a]	4	3	3.32
Box trainer model without specific knee characteristics	Level 1, ns	5	3	2.88

ns not significant
Level 1: high-level priority
[a]Items with $p < 0.001$

Table 2.6 Results of ranking exercises to train basic arthroscopic skills

Global exercises	Priority level	Rank	Median	Mean
Identification of structures and navigation with the arthroscope	Level 1[a]	1	5	4.46
Instrument handling	Level 1[a]	2	5	4.33
Preparation of patient and equipment	Level 1[a]	3	4	4.22
Detailed exercises				
Portal placement	Level 1[a]	1	5	4.66
Anatomical knowledge: Identification of different compartments, intercondylar notch including ACL and PCL, all important structures in the joint	Level 1[a]	2	5	4.6
Inspection with the arthroscope	Level 1[a]	3	5	4.54
Navigation by visualization of structures and probing them	Level 1[a]	4	5	4.41
Insertion arthroscope in anterolateral portal	Level 1[a]	5	5	4.37
Triangulation such as pick up a ball with a grasper, place the probe through a ring, and remove corpus liberum	Level 1[a]	6	5	4.26
Meniscectomy	Level 1[a]	7	4	4.22
Tissue manipulation	Level 1, ns	8	4	3.98
Meniscal suturing	Level 1, ns	9	4	3.76

ns not significant
Level 1: high-level priority
[a]Items with $p < 0.001$

the assumption of uniformity along the whole scale would be untenable (i.e., the distance between 1 and 2 is not as great as the distance between 4 and 5), as well as the assumption that different raters could agree on what single values really mean (i.e., 5 for rater A is not 5 for rater B).

In light of these considerations, we rather proceeded in the following way: (1) we counted the number of times each feature was ranked first, second, third, and so forth according to the *standard competition ranking* strategy; this is a strategy by which features that compare equal receive the same ranking number, and a gap is left in the ranking numbers (or *1224* strategy); (2) we normalized the sum of all rankings thus associated with each feature by the number of times that feature was actually evaluated; (3) finally, we created the final ranking of features by putting them in decreasing order from the feature with the lowest normalized rank sum to the feature with the highest sum.

Even with this method (let alone with arithmetic means), differences in ranking between single features are often negligible: this means that we cannot assert whether differences between features are due to chance (or to selection bias) or not, instead of being related to real differences in the perceived importance of respondents.

Thus, we also proceeded with a prioritization process and grouped the features in priority levels. To this aim, we counted the number of times each feature ranked in the first three positions for each respondent (*n*) and the number of times the same feature came in any other position (*m*). Then, we assigned each feature to the *high priority level* if *n* was greater than *m* and to the *low priority level* otherwise. Then, we also performed a chi-square test to evaluate the statistical significance of the difference between n and m, which in its turn could have been due to chance.

This created a feature prioritization process through which we assigned each feature to either two priority levels: higher priority (Level 1) and lower priority (Level 2). The reader should not consider features in Level 2 irrelevant, but only less relevant than those at Level 1 (on the other hand, absolute relevance is estimated with chi-square tests as reported above). However, some features could not be assigned to a priority level with statistical significance, as the repetition of this survey or involving different raters could lead to different assignment (no generalizability of results). Thus, we distinguish between Level 1 and Level 2 but we also indicate whether the assignment is significant, that is, independent of the specific sampling and consequently generalizable, or, conversely, likely due to chance. To this aim, we indicate if the assignment is significant (features with an asterisk *) or not (indicated with *ns*).

We believe that this way to proceed to analyses responses makes more sense than traditional mean-based ranking, as it allows interested researchers to detect what features should be really considered more important than the others, also in those surveys where most of the features were actually considered either relevant or very relevant, as it is in our case. Consequently, as a recommendation for decision-making, we consider priority levels first, in order to understand where to focus the main teaching efforts (high-level features first, then low level ones), and then take the single feature ranking to articulate more fine-grained interventions and teaching loads with respect to specific features that junior surgeons have to master.

2.3   Results of ESSKA Survey

A total of 195 orthopedic surgeons responded to the survey (response rate 19.5 %). Sixty-seven percent of the respondents had more than 10 years of personal experience in doing knee arthroscopy.

The number of knee arthroscopies performed by respondents in the last year was more than 400 for 11 % of the respondents, between 200 and 400 for 25 % of the respondents, between 50 and 200 for 46 % of the respondents, and less than 50 for the remaining 17 %.

A chi-square test of independence was performed to examine the difference in proportions between those who assigned a low importance to each item (response value 1 or 2) and those who assigned a high importance (response value 4 or 5). Except for triangulating the tip of the probe with a $0°$ scope, with a $70°$ scope, and box trainer model without specific knee characteristics ($p > 0.05$), the difference between these two proportions was significant for all variables ($p < 0.001$). This means that for these variables, the sample exhibited a strong polarization in their response considering the related skills "important to be mastered" in a statistically significant manner.

All general skills were considered important in equal manner by respondents as they were assigned to Level 1 of priority ($p < 0.001$) (Table 2.2).

The qualitative ranking method showed that anatomical knowledge was the most important skill, followed by triangulation and spatial perception (Table 2.2).

Even if sterility, knowledge of pathology, patient positioning, preparation before the operation, knowledge of equipment, and workup were ranked from 1 to 6, these specific skills were assigned to same level of priority (Level 1) ($p < 0.001$ and $p < 0.05$) (Table 2.3). Similarly, contact with patient and tissue manipulation (ranked from 7 to 8) were allocated to Level 1, but this result did not achieve the statistical significance (Table 2.3). Finally, the least important skills including hand positions and overall control in the operating room were allocated to an inferior priority level (Level 2) (Table 2.3).

Although precise portal placement was the most important feature investigating patient and tissue manipulation, features that were ranked from 1 to 7 were all assigned to high priority level (Level 1) (Table 2.4) whereas an inferior importance was observed for features ranked from 8 to 16 (Level 2) (Table 2.4).

In regard to the knowledge section, features ranked from 1 to 6 were perceived relevant in equal manner (Level 1, $p<0.001$) (Table 2.4). Features from 7 to 8 achieved the same level of importance without statistical significance (Level 1, ns). Knowledge of corpus liberum, of plica synovialis, and of Hoffa impingement (ranked from 9 to 11) was considered less relevant as they were assigned to Level 2 (Table 2.4). All features of navigation section were considered important in equal manner by respondents as they were allocated to same level of priority (Level 1) (Table 2.3).

2.4   Preferred Training Means

Vitale and coworkers (2007) created a survey to evaluate the methods by which orthopedic surgeons are trained in the skill of all-arthroscopic rotator cuff repair. When ranking the relative importance of resources in the training for all-arthroscopic repair, the overall Likert scale scores were highest for a sports medicine fellowship (3.49), hands-on instructional courses (3.33), and practice in an arthroscopy laboratory on cadaver specimens (3.22). Likert scores were lowest for residency training (2.02), practice on artificial shoulder models (2.13), and Internet resources (2.25). Safir and coworkers (2008) also suggested that high-fidelity simulation is preferred for training over low-fidelity benchtop models. Hui and coworkers (2013) found that higher-fidelity simulation models such as cadaveric specimens or the use of synthetic knees were preferred over lower-fidelity simulation models such as virtual reality simulators or benchtop models.

In the ESSKA survey, although cadaveric specimen was the top-ranked practice method to prepare a trainee before performing in the operating room, all practice methods were allocated to Level 1, and except for the box trainer model without specific knee characteristics, all items achieved the significance (Table 2.5).

All global exercises were considered relevant in equal manner by respondents as they were assigned to the highest level of priority (Level 1) (Table 2.6). Focusing on specific exercises,

although portal placement, identification of joint structures, and inspection with the arthroscope were ranked as the top three, all features achieved the same level of importance (Level 1) (Table 2.6).

2.5   Training to Become Competent

Arthroscopy is a core orthopedic skill and knee arthroscopy is the most common orthopedic procedure performed in the United States (Cullen et al. 2009). It is also the most common procedure recorded on case lists at the time of certification by the American Board of Orthopaedic Surgery (ABOS), with the numbers performed seen to be more than twice that of the second most common operation (Garrett et al. 2006). Review of the logbooks of candidates undertaking the oral component of the American Board exam also showed that five of the top eleven procedures involved arthroscopy. Knee arthroscopy has also been shown to constitute 30 % of all orthopedic procedures performed in Europe (Grechenig et al. 1999). Arthroscopy has certain specific technical requirements with a notable initial learning curve where the inexperienced surgeon requires greater supervision during a period of higher risk of iatrogenic injury as minimal access surgery requires different skills sets to open surgery (Allum 2002; Hanna et al. 1998). A study of senior orthopedic residents in the United States revealed that 68 % felt that there was inadequate time dedicated to training in arthroscopy in their program and 66 % did not feel as prepared in arthroscopic techniques as they did in open techniques (Hall et al. 2010).

The opinion of faculty was documented on how many repetitions an average resident needs in the operating room to become proficient in arthroscopic procedures. O'Neill and coworkers (2002) have presented quantitative numbers as a result of a questionnaire: on average, 50 (standard deviation (SD) 46) repetitions for partial medial meniscectomy, 61 (SD 53) for ACL reconstruction, 48 (SD 44) for diagnostic shoulder scope, and 58 (SD 56) for subacromial decompression. Leonard and coworkers (2007) stated that 41 diagnostic knee scopes (SD 18), 65 partial medial meniscectomies (SD 9), 88 partial lateral meniscectomies (SD 18), and 117 ACL reconstructions (SD 34) are required to achieve competency. A recent study by Koehler and coworkers indicated that more than 35 knee arthroscopies are required to demonstrate competency (Koehler and Nicandri 2013). The number of cases to become competent in hip arthroscopy was determined to be 30 and for arthroscopic Latarjet procedures was determined to be at least 15 cases (Castricini et al. 2013; Hoppe et al. 2014). An interesting result was that the absolute minimum number of repetitions needed to achieve proficiency was indicated to be 5–8 for any arthroscopic procedure (O'Neill et al. 2002).

2.6   Discussion

Patients are placing an additional demand of accountability on today's physicians and a surgeon must be capable of performing specific procedures in a safe and efficient manner such that the patient will not experience adverse consequence. A young surgeon should acquire specific skills before continuing training in the operating theatre. Even if this is a matter of concern, only few studies to date have tried to determine the relevance of skills that a simulator or training protocol should teach to young orthopedic surgeons.

2.7   Learning Objectives for Simulation Training

Knowledge on anatomy of the knee joint was ranked as the top one (Hui et al. 2013; Safir et al. 2008). This skill does not require actual instrument handling during training. As performing arthroscopy is largely dependent on visual cues received from the monitor, arthroscopic anatomy is suited to be taught outside the operating room, for example, using interactive e-learning modules that incorporate arthroscopic movies, pictures, and animated joint structures or using virtual reality simulators which also provide movies and

sometimes specific exercises focused on anatomy in combination with spatial perception (Obdeijn et al. 2013; Tuijthof et al. 2011). One other solution being explored is to use online simulators, where the program is held on a central server and where the simulator addresses those aspects of a surgical task that do not require a complex end-user controller that is expensive and fixed in one geographical location (Hurmusiadis et al. 2011). The other general skills do require actual instrument handling (Chami et al. 2008).

In general, the top five specific skills to be trained reflect the basic steps required to gain access and navigate into the joint. This seems straightforward as knowing your way in the joint will contribute to safe performance of the therapy.

2.8   Preferred Training Means

Questioning experts and residents what training means they prefer, cadaver courses are ranked number one followed by high-fidelity simulators (e.g., synthetic knee), virtual reality simulators, and box trainers.

Although arthroscopic simulators have the potential to enable residents and surgeons to further develop their skills in a safe environment, definitive conclusions on whether simulator training correlates to an improved arthroscopic skill set in the operating room are still not available (Frank et al. 2014). Moreover, as of now, none of the available trainers allows repetitive training of the most important skill: portal placement.

2.9   Training to Become Competent

Results of surveys have shown that at least up to eight patients are at risk at the start of each resident training program. An ideal situation is that before residents continue their training in the operating room, they should have achieved a competency level that guarantees safe arthroscopic treatment on their first patient. Logically, this should be one of the primary learning objectives for training arthroscopic skills in a simulated environment.

Bibliography

Allum R (2002) Complications of arthroscopy of the knee. J Bone Joint Surg Br 84(7):937–945, available from: PM:12358382

Biggs J (2003) Constructing learning by aligning teaching: constructive alignment. In: Biggs J (ed) Teaching for quality learning at university, 2nd edn. Open University Press, Berkshire, pp 11–33

Castricini R, De BM, Orlando N, Rocchi M, Zini R, Pirani P (2013) Arthroscopic Latarjet procedure: analysis of the learning curve. Musculoskelet Surg 97(Suppl 1):93–98, available from: PM:23588833

Chami G, Ward JW, Phillips R, Sherman KP (2008) Haptic feedback can provide an objective assessment of arthroscopic skills. Clin Orthop Relat Res 466(4):963–968, available from: PM:18213507

Cullen KA, Hall MJ, Golosinskiy A (2009) Ambulatory surgery in the United States, 2006. Natl Health Stat Report (11) January 28:1–25 available from: PM:19294964

Frank RM, Erickson B, Frank JM, Bush-Joseph CA, Bach BR Jr, Cole BJ, Romeo AA, Provencher MT, Verma NN (2014) Utility of modern arthroscopic simulator training models. Arthroscopy 30(1):121–133, available from: PM:24290789

Garrett WE Jr, Swiontkowski MF, Weinstein JN, Callaghan J, Rosier RN, Berry DJ, Harrast J, Derosa GP (2006) American Board of Orthopaedic Surgery Practice of the Orthopaedic Surgeon: Part-II, certification examination case mix. J Bone Joint Surg Am 88(3):660–667, available from: PM:16510834

Grechenig W, Fellinger M, Fankhauser F, Weiglein AH (1999) The Graz learning and training model for arthroscopic surgery. Surg Radiol Anat 21(5):347–350, available from: PM:10635100

Hall MP, Kaplan KM, Gorczynski CT, Zuckerman JD, Rosen JE (2010) Assessment of arthroscopic training in U.S. orthopedic surgery residency programs–a resident self-assessment. Bull NYU Hosp Jt Dis 68(1): 5–10, available from: PM:20345354

Hanna GB, Shimi SM, Cuschieri A (1998) Randomised study of influence of two-dimensional versus three-dimensional imaging on performance of laparoscopic cholecystectomy. Lancet 351(9098):248–251, available from: PM:9457094

Hoppe DJ, de SD, Simunovic N, Bhandari M, Safran MR, Larson CM, Ayeni OR (2014) The learning curve for hip arthroscopy: a systematic review. Arthroscopy 30:389–397, available from: PM:24461140

Hui Y, Safir O, Dubrowski A, Carnahan H (2013) What skills should simulation training in arthroscopy teach residents? A focus on resident input. Int J Comput Assist Radiol Surg 8:945–953, available from: PM:23535939

Hurmusiadis V, Rhode K, Schaeffter T, Sherman K (2011) Virtual arthroscopy trainer for minimally invasive surgery. Stud Health Technol Inform 163:236–238, available from: PM:21335795

Koehler RJ, Nicandri GT (2013) Using the arthroscopic surgery skill evaluation tool as a pass-fail examination. J Bone Joint Surg Am 95(23):e1871–e1876, available from: PM:24306710

Leonard M, Kennedy J, Kiely P, Murphy P (2007) Knee arthroscopy: how much training is necessary? A cross-sectional study. Eur J Orthop Surg Traumatol 17:359–362

O'Neill PJ, Cosgarea AJ, Freedman JA, Queale WS, McFarland EG (2002) Arthroscopic proficiency: a survey of orthopaedic sports medicine fellowship directors and orthopaedic surgery department chairs. Arthroscopy 18(7):795–800, available from: PM:12209439

Obdeijn MC, Bavinck N, Mathoulin C, van der Horst CM, Schijven MP, Tuijthof GJ (2013) Education in wrist arthroscopy: past, present and future. Knee Surg Sports Traumatol Arthrosc. available from: PM:23835770

Safir O, Dubrowski A, Mirsky L, Lin C, Backstein D, Carnahan A (2008) What skills should simulation training in arthroscopy teach residents? Int J Comput Assist Radiol Surg 3(5):433–437

Tuijthof GJ, Visser P, Sierevelt IN, van Dijk CN, Kerkhoffs GM (2011) Does perception of usefulness of arthroscopic simulators differ with levels of experience? Clin Orthop Relat Res 469:1701–1708, available from: PM:21290203

Vitale MA, Kleweno CP, Jacir AM, Levine WN, Bigliani LU, Ahmad CS (2007) Training resources in arthroscopic rotator cuff repair. J Bone Joint Surg Am 89(6):1393–1398, available from: PM:17545443

Theory on Psychomotor Learning Applied to Arthroscopy

3

John J. van den Dobbelsteen, Mustafa Karahan, and Umut Akgün

"I hear and I forget. I see, I remember. I do, I understand." – Confucius

Take-Home Messages

- Learning to use arthroscopic instruments involves minimization of predicted and actual sensory information by tuning the internal models in our brain that represent the tasks at hand.
- As all individuals demonstrate differences in innate arthroscopic skills, the training period should vary in order to allow all trainees to achieve a preset competency level.
- Exposure to many different conditions in a training program facilitates skills learning.
- A perfect teacher is not the one who has the best ability to perform a specific motor skill but the one who has the ability to transfer a skill to a student.
- Developing "ideal" training programs for basic part task arthroscopic skills is needed to complement current residency curricula

J.J. van den Dobbelsteen (✉)
Department of Biomechanical Engineering,
Delft University of Technology,
Delft, The Netherlands
e-mail: J.J.vandenDobbelsteen@tudelft.nl

M. Karahan • U. Akgün
Department of Orthopedics and Traumatology,
Acibadem University School of Medicine,
Istanbul, Turkey
e-mail: drmustafakarahan@gmail.com;
umut.akgun@acibadem.edu.tr

3.1 Definitions

Sensorimotor relates to activity involving both sensory and motor pathways of the nerves (Oxford English Dictionary 2014).

(Psycho)motor skill is the potential to produce voluntary muscular movements after practice (Kaufman et al. 1987; Oxford English Dictionary 2014).

Psychomotor learning is an interaction between cognitive functions and physical activities with the emphasis on learning coordinated activity involving the arms, hands, fingers, and feet.

Efference copy is an internal copy of an outflowing, movement-producing signal generated by our human motor system (Kawato 1999; Wolpert and Miall 1996).

Internal model is a postulated neural process that simulates the response of the motor system in order to estimate the outcome of a motor command (Kawato 1999; Wolpert and Miall 1996).

3.2 Introduction

This chapter is highly interesting as it brings together theories from different fields – i.e. neuroscience, education, and arthroscopy – which combination gives insights in human performance capabilities when interacting with the environment and more specifically effectively training arthroscopic skills, the title of this book.

M. Karahan et al. (eds.), *Effective Training of Arthroscopic Skills*,
DOI 10.1007/978-3-662-44943-1_3, © ESSKA 2015

Section A describes the state of the art on senso-rimotor learning from a neuroscience perspective, whereas Section B discusses psychomotor skills in arthroscopic training through the science of learning.

3.3 Section A: Sensorimotor Learning from Neuroscientific Perspective

The range and complexity of the tasks involved in arthroscopy are impressive but even more so is the capacity of humans to learn the variety of precise and delicate motor skills needed to successfully perform these operative procedures (Kaufman et al. 1987). Arthroscopic instruments introduce changes in the relationship between the movements of the surgeons' hand and the tip of the instrument. The use of arthroscopic instruments challenges the operators' sensorimotor abilities, by requesting efficient gathering of the often limited and distorted sensory information and by requesting the implementation of adaptive mechanisms to perform instrument handling. Mastery of instrument handling implies that one is able to account for complex transformations, as is, for example, needed to cope with the disturbed eye-hand coordination (Miller 1985) and the uncertainties about task-relevant information when planning the movements.

When we use novel tools in everyday life, we are exposed to a new mechanical environment. The tools initially perturb our movements, but after practice, we are again able to process a certain input (the sensory information provided by our sensor organs – eyes, proprioception) to obtain the desired output (the movement of the tip of the instrument). Learning of surgical skills can be thought of as the process of mastering and adapting such sensorimotor transformations. Depending on the complexity of the transformations, this may take several hundred movements. This is reflected in the prolonged learning curves for the minimally invasive techniques, in comparison to the time needed to acquire the skills for open surgery (Atesok et al. 2012; Megali et al. 2005).

In the past decade, there have been substantial advances in our understanding of how we learn (psycho)motor skills, with models emerging from computational approaches to movement science. The following is a discussion of the main concepts for our understanding of learning surgical motor skills:

Internal models
Sensory weighting
Structural and parametric learning

These concepts will be applied to understand and explain the, often limited, transfer of learning from the training situation to the real performance in the operating room.

3.3.1 Internal Models

It is generally believed that the process of learning skilled control relies on the acquisition of models of both our own body and the instruments we interact with (Davidson and Wolpert 2003; Flanagan et al. 2003). Learning to control a new instrument (i.e., act in a novel environment) produces an "internal model" that represents the sensorimotor transformations involved in the use of the instrument. Two main classes of internal models are being distinguished: forward models and inverse models. Here, we describe how these two fundamental concepts of motor control are related to learning to handle arthroscopic instruments.

Forward internal models describe the causal relationship between our interactions with the instrument and the environment and the sensory feedback that will result from these interactions (Wolpert and Miall 1996).

In particular, they allow us to predict the sensory consequences of our actions on the basis of a copy of the motor command (i.e., efference copy) that is send to our motor system (Fig. 3.1). These predictions are essential for acquiring a training signal when learning a new task. This is elucidated with one aspect of performing an arthroscopic procedure: the scaling of visual

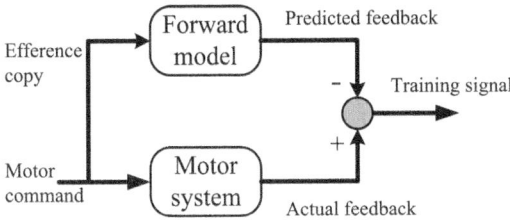

Fig. 3.1 Forward models are necessary for learning. A copy of the motor command is used to predict the sensory feedback. The prediction is compared to the actual feedback. A discrepancy in the sensory signals can be used for training

motion of the instruments seen via the two-dimensional monitor. The arthroscopic image is a zoomed-in two-dimensional projection of the surgical area, for which the exact zoomed-in scale factor is initially unknown to the trainee. As a consequence, the predicted visual motion of the instrument tip is likely to be underestimated: one moves too far. This difference between the predicted and the actual sensory information results in an error that can be used as a training signal to update the internal model (Fig. 3.1). In a subsequent repetition of this aspect, the error is likely to be smaller by generating an adapted motor command, which is sent to the involved muscles.

The second group of internal models that are relevant for understanding motor learning are known as inverse models. These models perform the opposite transformation in that they obtain the required motor command from the desired sensory consequences. Thus, when the task is to reach a visual location as seen on the monitor, one needs to compute the required hand movement in order to achieve this desired state. In the above-presented example, where the actual visual motion on the monitor screen was larger than intended, the thus generated error signal can also be used to update the inverse model and by that induce learning.

In summary, learning to use arthroscopic instruments involves both building up inverse models to control the instrument and forward models for predicting the consequences of this control. Discrepancies between predicted and actual sensory information generate an error signal that is a prerequisite for learning.

3.3.2 Sensory Weighting

The accuracy of the error signals generated with help of forward models not only depends on the accuracy of the predicted feedback but also on the accuracy of our estimate of the actual sensory information. The signals obtained from our sensors are disturbed by internal noise (i.e., in the neural transmission). However, when we have various sources of information available, then these can be optimally combined to achieve estimates that reduce the effects of noise (van Beers 2009). For instance, when moving the hand to a visual target, the location of the target and the location of the hand need to be to be determined. Both visual information and proprioceptive information contribute to estimations of the positions of the target and the hand. When information is available in both modalities, we combine these sources of information into one coherent idea of where objects are relative to ourselves.

This integration process also needs to take into account the disturbances in sensory information inflicted by external objects, such as the surgical instruments and the operative environment. In the case of arthroscopic procedures, the sensory information is often limited and distorted. Altered 30° viewing angle of the arthroscope makes that the visual and proprioceptive modalities are no longer aligned. Friction and reaction forces of the manipulated tissue often disturb the forces experienced at the handle of the instruments. Especially in the inexperienced trainees, this induces movement inaccuracy and variability.

The ability of humans to compensate for such disturbances is a well-studied phenomenon. In a wide range of tasks, it has been found that humans are still able to perform well by optimally combining sensory cues. For instance, it has been shown that the optimal use of unaligned sensory information can limit movement errors in the absence of vision (Smeets et al. 2006). These studies show that when we have knowledge about the reliability of our sensory information, we can combine different modalities together in a statistically optimal manner. Depending on the reliability of the information, different weights are assigned to the sensory signals when they are combined. Therefore, one important aspect of training arthroscopic skills may be sufficient exposure to the variable conditions that can be encountered. This enables the trainee to come to an estimate of the reliability of the sensory information that is available in the procedures. The variable conditions include different handling instruments form different companies, anatomic variations of human joints, variation in pathologies (e.g., meniscal tears), and different disturbance conditions (e.g., bleedings). An advantage of offering many variable conditions is that trainees remain motivated as they need to deal with new situations in subsequent training sessions.

The idea arises that the crucial difficulties in arthroscopic skills are much more related to a lack of experience with the large variety of disturbing sensations as opposed to a lack of experience with instrument-tissue interaction per se. This is supported by a study of Bholat and coworkers (1999) that shows that, without vision, both expert surgeons and novices are able to correctly identify object properties when using minimally invasive instruments. In this study, the movements of the instruments were not constrained so that no other external objects could affect the sensations of the subjects. Therefore, the substantial performance differences between experts and novices in arthroscopy presumably only arise, because experts are better able to discard the disturbing sensations due to their larger experience with various instruments and the compact intra-articular operative environments. As all individuals demonstrate differences in innate arthroscopic skills, the training period should vary in order to allow all trainees to achieve a preset competency level (Alvand et al. 2011; Kaufman et al. 1987).

3.3.3 Structural and Parametric Learning

Once we have learned a motor skill, such as moving arthroscopic instruments under highly zoomed-in viewing conditions, we can rapidly generalize to other surgical situations in which the field of view is scaled and movements are visually amplified, even though the scaling factor may differ. Such fast learning can presumably be accomplished by making small adjustments to the parameters of an existing internal model. This parametric learning implies that the model is already available and that only the proper parameters need to be adapted. Such adaptive learning has been reported in a large variety of motor tasks (Shadmehr et al. 2010).

One difficulty with learning to control a new instrument is that the physical properties of the instrument are initially unknown and need to be characterized first in the process of building up an internal model. An important part of this learning process is identifying the relevant inputs and outputs of the system and the transformations that define the relationship between them. Through experience with many comparable instruments, one might discover the general form of the transformations for a certain type of instrument (Braun et al. 2010). For instance, the consequence of operating through small incisions in the skin is that the movement of the hand is opposite to the desired motion of the effective part of the instrument (fulcrum effect). Such complex transformations are in essence what is learned in structural learning, whereas subsequent parametric learning would involve selecting the proper parameters for the currently used instrument (i.e., the scaling of the movements).

Evidence for structural learning comes from a study of Braun and coworkers (2009). In a series of experiments, they exposed human subjects to rotary visuomotor transformations in different virtual reality environments. The parameters of these transformations (i.e., the direction and angle of rotation) were varied randomly over many trials, but the structure of the transformation (i.e., the presence of a rotation) was always the same. Because subjects showed faster learning of such transformations after random training, they must have learned much more than the average mapping as one would expect for simple parametric learning.

Enhancement of structural learning may also be achieved by means of providing additional information about the interactions of the instruments with the environment and therefore increasing the transparency of the transformations.

For instance, previous research has shown that providing information about the orientation of the tip of the instrument improves performance in tasks performed with a minimally invasive simulator (Wentink et al. 2002). Horeman and coworkers (2012) showed that continuous visual information about exerted forces reduced the magnitude of forces used in manipulating minimally invasive instruments (see also Chap. 9). However, retention of learning with such substituted feedback is generally low.

Sülzenbrück and Heuer (2012) demonstrate that visual feedback that enhances mechanical transparency can have opposite effects on learning. It is likely that the visual feedback reduces the need to build up an accurate internal model of the instrument interactions as evidenced by the lack of improvement once the visual feedback is removed. Alternatively, substituted sensory feedback, like visual information that represents exerted forces (e.g., cognitive representations), may require additional transformations to update internal models relevant for force control. In the study of Horeman and coworkers (2012), the visual information needs to be transformed into an error signal that is suitable to train the models of the dynamics of the task. Possibly, it is more beneficial to provide error signals within the sensory modality that is relevant for the task.

In summary, training of arthroscopic skills benefits most from approaches that induce learning of the general structure of the task, the characteristics of the transformations imposed by the arthroscopic instruments. Structural learning is mostly facilitated by exposure to a variety of tasks that share this common structure. Substituted feedback enhances the transparency of the transformations and can support performance but may be less efficient for building up new internal models.

3.3.4 Transfer of Learning

In the above, we have discussed how structural learning could provide a mechanism for transfer of learning between tasks with the same task structure. Building up experience in one or more tasks often enables one to subsequently learn related tasks more rapidly. "Transfer of learning" has been demonstrated for various motor tasks (Braun et al. 2009; Seidler 2007). Unfortunately, there is still insufficient evidence for transfer of skills from surgical training programs to in vivo performance in the operating room (Modi et al. 2010; Slade Shantz et al. 2014). In surgical training often simulators, e.g., computer-controlled virtual environments, are employed as they allow precise control of the task parameters and assessment of specific performance measurements (Chap. 5). In general, these simulators mimic only part of a surgical procedure. So far, results suggest that simulator training only improves performance in the same task in the same simulator (Strom et al. 2004).

The lack of transfer can partly be explained by our ability to control a large variety of instruments with different physical characteristics. When we use different instruments, the context of our movement changes in a discrete manner. For dexterous control of the instruments, we must select the appropriate internal model on the basis of contextual cues (Fig. 3.2). However, a perfect match is rarely found, because the instrument properties may fluctuate over time (e.g., due to wear, friction), and the exact environmental conditions (e.g., the patient) may never have been encountered.

Therefore, just as we need to combine sensory information to optimally estimate our current state, we need to derive models from combinations of previously experienced situations. The central idea is that when we encounter novel situations, with unknown dynamics, we weigh the outputs of several internal models selected on the basis of sensory information, for appropriate performance (Fig. 3.2).

Crucial in the above-proposed scheme is that skilled manipulation in untrained situations requires previous exposure to many comparable contexts with various dynamics (Kording and Wolpert 2004; Wolpert and Ghahramani 2000). In contrast, an often-adopted solution in surgical training simulators is to create conditions in which the training context mimics the real

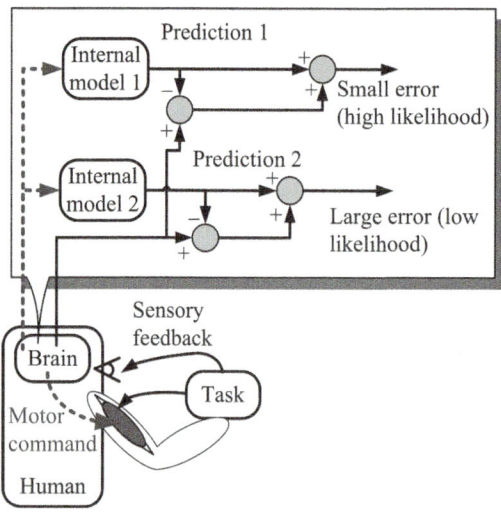

Fig. 3.2 The internal model is chosen that is most likely to predict the smallest estimation error

3.4 Section B: Psychomotor Learning from Educational Perspective

Learning and teaching have a very old history. Written records showed that ancestors of formal education were seen in Egypt around 500 B.C (Tokuhama-Espinosa 2010). Through the human history, educators tried to develop better ways of teaching. In 1956, Benjamin Bloom and a group of educational psychologists developed a classification of educational objectives known as "Bloom's Taxonomy" (Bloom et al. 1956).

Taxonomy divides educational objectives into three domains: cognitive (Fig. 3.3a), affective (Fig. 3.3b), and psychomotor. Within the domains, learning at the higher levels is dependent on having attained prerequisite knowledge and skills at lower levels. Bloom's Taxonomy guides educators to focus on all three domains, creating a holistic form of education.

Benjamin Bloom has completed his work on cognitive and affective domains, but never completed the psychomotor domain. Dave was the first to suggested simple form of the psychomotor domain in 1970 (Dave 1970) and underlined the significant role of "imitation" in psychomotor learning (Fig. 3.3c). In the 1990s, Anderson and coworkers updated the taxonomy to reflect today's educational systems (Fig. 3.3d) (Anderson et al. 2001). Examples of psychomotor skills learning in daily life include driving a car, throwing a ball, and playing a musical instrument.

As indicated in Section A, the psychomotor domain of learning is not explained by pure knowledge or experience (Rovai et al. 2009) but focuses on sensorimotor skill development involving parameters such as speed, accuracy, and grace of movement and dexterity (Anderson et al. 2001; Rovai et al. 2009). Initially, these manual tasks can be simple such as throwing a ball but can become complicated such as arthroscopic surgery. As they increase in complexity, the amount of overall skills needed to execute the task also increases. That is why psychomotor learning cannot be isolated from the cognitive domain. One should have sufficient

performance context as closely as possible and, more importantly, always with the same physical properties. The drawback of this approach is reflected in the lack of transfer of learning from one simulator to another. Albeit similar, the properties of the simulated may slightly differ so that a less effective internal model is selected.

The idea emerges that the broad repertoire of motor skills needed in the operating room can be more effectively learned when being trained in much more variable environmental conditions using a diversity of instruments. From a pragmatic perspective, such an approach also reduces the need to recreate real situations in the training setting which is probably also more cost-effective. The validity of this perspective for training of arthroscopy is illustrated by studies that compare the performance of expert surgeons and trainees on novel surgical trainers. Although expert surgeons generally display better performance than novices, the performance of experts improves with practice, as well as that of novices (Chap. 7) (Pedowltz et al. 2002, Tuijthof et al. 2011). Presumably, the learning curves of the experts reflect further optimization in the weighting process based on the sensory information that is currently experienced in this novel situation.

Fig. 3.3 (**a**) Levels of cognitive domain of Taxonomy in the 1950s (Bloom et al. 1956). (**b**) Levels of affective domain of Taxonomy in the 1950s (Bloom et al. 1956). (**c**) Levels of psychomotor domain of Taxonomy in the 1970s (Dave 1970). (**d**) Levels of Taxonomy updated by Anderson and coworkers in the 1990s (Anderson et al. 2001)

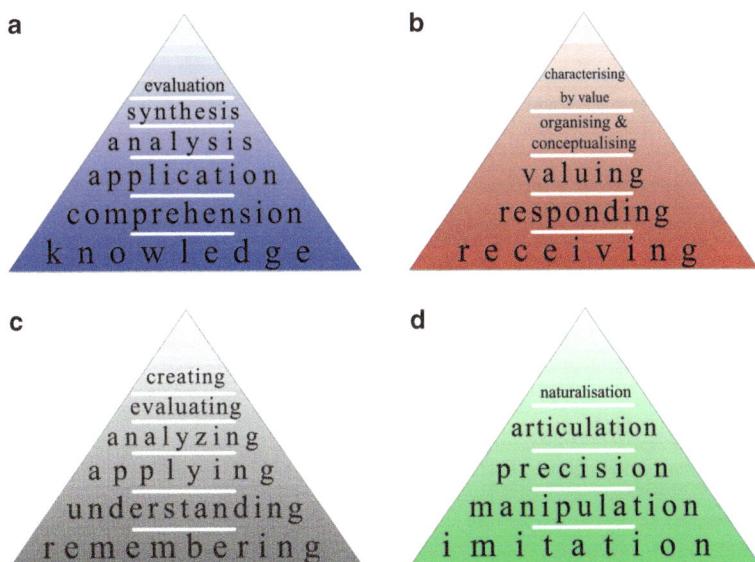

theoretical information about the skill that is going to be trained but also know what type of learning style in order to design an "ideal" training program to learn arthroscopic skills. In the remainder, learning styles, psychomotor acquisition models, feedback, and other elements are discussed that need to be taken into account when designing such an "ideal" training program.

3.4.1 Learning Styles

Individuals have different ways of learning. In adult learners, three types of learning styles are defined: visual, auditory and kinesthetic learners, which make up around 65, 30, and 5 % of the population, respectively (Dankelman et al. 2005). Visual learners need slide presentations, pictures, flow charts, videos, and handouts. In society, they will tend to be the most effective in written communication and symbol manipulation (Dankelman et al. 2005). Dialogues, discussions, and debates are the main tools for auditory learners, who may be sophisticated speakers. Kinesthetic learners learn effectively through touch, movement, and space; they learn skills by imitation and practice. They benefit

highly from games and hands-on training sessions. A quick way to determine what learning style you have is to follow this link to the VARK-Learn questionnaire (www.vark-learn. com) (Kim et al. 2013). Training techniques and teaching programs should be designed such to accommodate the three learning styles (Windsor et al. 2008).

Learning styles of adults are also related with intelligence of the individuals. Gardner developed multiple intelligence theory to define a relation with the learning styles of individuals (Gardner 2011). According to his theory, intelligence of trainees is classified into nine categories (Table 3.1). Each person has these intelligences; however, their ratios vary from one to another. Ratios of these intelligences in a person can also change over time, because of environmental factors. This is a major obstacle in front of when trying to design an "ideal" arthroscopic teaching program.

To accommodate the learning style of individuals in respect to their intelligences, a pre-course evaluation would be useful. MIDAS stands for Multiple Intelligences Developmental Assessment Scale (www.miresearch.org) that is a self-administered questionnaire to define the learning styles of individuals before starting a

Table 3.1 Details of the Gardner's multiple intelligences (Gardner 2011)

Multiple intelligence type	Incorporated into subject matter	Way of demonstrating understanding
Linguistic	Books, stories, speeches, author visits	Writing stories, scripts, storytelling
Logical	Exercises, drills, problem solving	Calculating, theorizing, demonstrating, computer programming
Musical	Tapes, CDs, concert going	Performing, singing, playing, composing
Visual-spatial	Posters, art work, slides, charts, graphs, videos, museum visits	Drawing, illustrating, collage making, photography
Bodily kinesthetic	Movies, animations, exercises, physicalizing concepts	Dance recital, athletic performance or composition
Interpersonal	Teams, group work, specialist roles	Debates, panels, group work
Intrapersonal	Reflection time, meditation exercises	Journals, diaries, habits, personal growth
Naturalist	Aquariums, pets, farm, nature walks, museum visits	Collecting, classifying, caring for animals and nature
Existential	Working on causes, charity work	Community service

training program (Shearer 1998). By using MIDAS, trainees' primary, secondary, and tertiary intelligences can be identified prior to a course; in the long run, this can be helpful to design specific training programs, perhaps even per learning style. In a previous study among surgeons, it was shown that trainees with a primary "bodily kinesthetic" intelligence were the best performers in laparoscopic tasks (Windsor et al. 2008). Thus, knowing once learning style is a prerequisite for both trainee and teacher to achieve an optimal learning experience.

3.4.2 Psychomotor Learning Education Models

Fitts and Posner proposed a three-stage model of learning psychomotor skill (Fitts and Posner 1967):

Cognitive Stage
In the cognitive stage, tasks are well defined, and appropriate consecutive actions are listed needed to accomplish the task goals. This stage usually interacts with the knowledge of the trainee. In other words, one must have enough theoretical information to complete the cognitive stage. Characteristic of this stage is that the trainee must think about the execution of each action before doing so, which results in slow and intermittent actions.

Associative Stage
Once the cognitive stage is accomplished, the trainee can focus on the details of the actions to achieve task completion. In this transient associative stage, the required actions are split into simple sensorimotor skills, and smooth transition between these skills is exercised. This results in a decrease of the time consumed for thinking about the action, but actions are not fluent yet.

Autonomic Stage
The final stage is the autonomous stage, in which the trainee can perform the necessary sensorimotor skills fluently and completes predefined task goals in an optimal or efficient manner. Thus, the trainee does not need to spend time to think about the action and demonstrate a fluent skill.

A characteristic feature of this three-stage model is that the initial stages have a rapid progression whereas slowly progress to the autonomic stage. Simpson described more detailed stages of psychomotor learning connected to teaching strategies (Simpson 1972). This psychomotor learning model consists of (1) perception, (2) ability to perform a specific task by the guidance of a supervisor, (3) ability to perform a specific task without supervision, (4) ability to perform a complex pattern of simple tasks, (5) ability to respond to new situations by altering the action plan, and (6) ability to develop new action plans. This model represents the transformation of a rookie to a pro, as can also be seen in the

Global Rating Scales scoring forms (Appendices 13A-E). According to Van Merriënboer and coworkers, one should be careful not to assume that learning of a complex task is the sum of part tasks, because it also includes the ability to coordinate and integrate those parts (Merrienboer et al. 2002). This latter is basically already applied in the residency curricula of arthroscopy, as training in the operating room requires this form of integration, which is reflected in the holistic type of performance monitoring (Chap. 14). However, part task training is especially needed, when certain actions need to be automated. This is where basic skills training in simulated environments can play a central role in increasing learning efficiency of psychomotor skills.

3.4.3 Preconditions for a Training Program of Basic Arthroscopic Skills

In today's surgical education, most of the endoscopic skills are practiced on real patients. Studies showed that a surgeon may need 15–100 cases to reach proficiency which may take quite a time on clinical setup (American Board of Internal Medicine 1991; Eversbusch and Grantcharov 2004; Hawes et al. 1986; Hoppe et al. 2014; O'Neill et al. 2002). The difficulty of teaching in a clinical setup as it resembles the highest level of task complexity forced medical educators to seek different and effective training tools. Until recently, the abovementioned basic skills training has not been given a lot of attention. That is why it will have the focus in the remainder of this section. Several important preconditions are discussed that need to be taken into account when design the "ideal" basic training program.

In other fields that require psychomotor skills training such as sports and playing a music instruments, the abovementioned theories have been used to design different educational programs. The general approach has been to divide a complex task into basic pat tasks. For example, when training basketball players, basic skills such as dribbling and passing are thought before full court playing. In archery, one must exercise

inspiration techniques and hand-eye coordination before shooting. Another program involving this kind of stepped skill teaching has been successfully used in music students (Neiman 1989).

3.4.4 Define Basic Skills

Nowadays, information on the science of learning and education gradually is being applied in residency training. To use or adapt previous studies and knowledge about psychomotor learning to arthroscopic training, a first crucial step would be the unambiguous definition of the basic skills that is needed for the arthroscopic tasks. In the current literature, basic skills are not standardized; many others can be added. In a different study, Suksudaj and coworkers tested different psychomotor skills and showed that tracing is an important basic skill among dental students, which is correlated with performances (Suksudaj et al. 2012). Neequaye and coworkers showed basic components of endovascular surgical procedures (Neequaye et al. 2007). Chapter 2 presents data that can be used to fulfill this precondition for arthroscopy as well. When defining such basic skills, one must consider the basic components of endoscopic surgery. The main differences between endoscopic surgeries and open surgeries are loss of binocularity, loss of tactile feedback, the *fulcrum effect* of portals (as mentioned in Section A), and the need for triangulation. Two-dimensional monitors are used in endoscopic surgeries, and this leads to the loss of binocularity. Loss of binocularity means that you lose substantial part of your depth perception. Tactile feedback is a very important cue in open surgery as surgeons use it to discriminate between normal and pathologic tissues. During endoscopic surgeries, tactile feedback is substantially decreased because of the instruments such as probes that act as interface between the hand of the surgeon and the tissue. This implies that surgeons need to rely more on the visual impression behavior of tissue when probing. A characteristic of experienced endoscopic surgeons is their ability of anticipation to this new environment to cope with the lost or disturbed cues.

The last important difference, the *fulcrum effect*, is caused by the portal dependency in endoscopic surgeries (Gallagher et al. 2009). This reverse relation causes a visual proprioceptive conflict for the surgeon's brain (Gallagher et al. 2005). As this effect is so different from interactions with our environment in daily lives, this conflict consumes a significant time for the surgeon to adapt. Bilateralism and triangulation are helpful to overcome the fulcrum effect.

The abovementioned basic skills can be exercised in training simulators as presented in Chaps. 3, 4, and 5. So the training means are available, the next step would to design validated exercises to train them and to extend the arthroscopic curriculum with these exercises to improve the residents' performances and achieve efficient learning.

3.5   Example of a Basic Skill Course

Karahan and coworkers are among the first to propose such a basic skills training program, which has been validated. The program consists of a 2-day course consisting of six modules (Unalan et al. 2010):

1. Interactive presentations about arthroscopic technology and basic knee pathologies.
2. Video presentations of basic arthroscopic procedures.
3. Basic motor skill exercises such as triangulation; depth are shown in (Chap. 6, Fig. 6.1).
4. Triangulation exercises on dry knee joint models or virtual reality simulators.
5. Wet lab exercises on a cow knee (Chap. 5), which is mainly designed to mimic a real arthroscopic procedure.
6. The knot station, in which all participants can train surgical knot tying again on a very basic model.

In their studies, Karahan and coworkers and Unalan and coworkers showed that experienced surgeons outperform the novices in reaction time and double-arm coordination time when executing the basic skills exercises of Module 3 (Karahan et al. 2009; Unalan et al. 2010). This is in line with the theory that assumes that skill can be explained as the ability to perform a specific task with less energy and time (Straub and Terrace 1981).

3.6   Additional Points of Attention

When designing a basic skill training program, other elements of psychomotor learning should also be considered. Training time or the number of training sets in order to achieve proficiency on a skill can vary from one surgeon to another. For example, Eversbusch and Grantcharov concluded that ten repetitions on a gastrointestinal simulator would be enough to acquire basic skills (Eversbusch and Grantcharov 2004). In a different study, Unalan and coworkers as well as Verdaasdonk and coworkers used ten repetitions on basic motor skill training instruments to achieve the plateau in the learning curve (Unalan et al. 2010; Verdaasdonk et al. 2007). An average number of repetitions on a specific training instrument should be defined before organizing a training program.

Another important element is the loss of a gained skill. Gallagher and coworkers showed that 2 weeks of no use will cause loss of recently acquired skills (Gallagher et al. 2012), whereas Gomoll and coworkers showed that continued training indeed maintained skill proficiency over a period of 3 years (Gomoll et al. 2008). Any training program should be followed by a practicing session within weeks in order to reinforce the skill acquisition.

Feedback is another important point in psychomotor learning. Closed-loop theory points out that feedbacks are important in skill acquisition. Trainees receiving verbal feedback while performing a task do better than the ones who do not receive that (Adams 1971). This finding is supported in various other studies in which structured feedback was compared with no additional feedback during endoscopic surgery by decreased errors and improved learning curves of the feedback groups (Boyle et al. 2011; Harewood et al. 2008; O'Connor et al. 2008; Triano et al. 2006). Live feedback during skill teaching may provide a better learning environment. Consequently, arthroscopic training programs should include interactive sessions with real-time feedback mechanisms.

3.7   Discussion

Although the precise nature of the mechanisms involved in learning arthroscopic techniques are at this point still largely unknown, the hypothetical constructs discussed in the current chapter provide a framework for our thinking about training programs for arthroscopic surgeons. The importance of such a methodical approach is obvious when one considers the variations in the acquisition of surgical skills among residents (Alvand et al. 2011). Prior to a course or training program, trainees can be assessed on their initial skills levels with instruments for dexterity tests and on their learning style with online questionnaires. Both tests can be done within minute and provide the teachers valuable information to adapt to the trainee's levels and enhance transfer of knowledge and experience.

Skills training programs should focus on facilitating the buildup of internal models of the arthroscopic instruments and the environment they interact with – which are the human joints. The approach of using training tools, such as instruments virtual reality training simulators, will be useful to automate certain surgical actions. However, the current absence of sufficient clinical variation in these simulators makes them insufficient to mimic actual procedures. Experiencing task variation will enhance learning of the structure of the task as opposed to merely learning one set of parameter values that only applies for a specific training condition. Therefore, it is of much more importance to ensure that the variability in training tools and

tasks captures the subtle but high variability of sensory information that is encountered in the real procedures. This is, for example, the case in the presented 2-day basic arthroscopy course.

A well-designed adult teaching program should cover all these needs; one should not forget that competent teachers are equally important to complete an "ideal" teaching program. A perfect teacher is not the one who has the best ability to perform a specific motor skill but the one who has the ability to transfer that skill to a student.

In conclusion, including psychomotor learning theory into our daily training grounds, teaching skills will be more efficient and effective. As much as it seems as if it is "other people's ball field," theory on learning is for us orthopedic surgeons a primary concern and should be applied on a day-to-day basis. Only then we will become true teachers.

Bibliography

Adams JA (1971) A closed-loop theory of motor learning. J Mot Behav 3(2):111–149, available from: PM:15155169

Allum R (2002) Complications of arthroscopy of the knee. J Bone Joint Surg Br 84(7):937–945, available from: PM:12358382

Alvand A, Auplish S, Gill H, Rees J (2011) Innate arthroscopic skills in medical students and variation in learning curves. J Bone Joint Surg Am 93(19):e115–e119, available from: PM:22005876

American Board of Internal Medicine (1991) Guide to evaluation of residents in internal medicine, 1991–1992. American Board of Internal Medicine, Philadelphia

Amrein A, Berliner D (2002) High-stakes testing & student learning. Educ Policy Anal Arch 10:18

Anderson LW, Kratwohl DR, Airasian PW, Cruikshank KA, Mayer RE, Pintrich PR, Raths J, Wittrock MC (2001) A taxonomy for learning, teaching, and assessing: a revision of Bloom's taxonomy of educational objectives. Pearson, Allyn & Bacon, New York

Atesok K, Mabrey JD, Jazrawi LM, Egol KA (2012) Surgical simulation in orthopaedic skills training. J Am Acad Orthop Surg 20(7):410–422, available from: PM:22751160

Awad SS, Fagan SP, Bellows C, Albo D, Green-Rashad B, De la Garza M, Berger DH (2005) Bridging the communication gap in the operating room with medical team training. Am J Surg 190(5):770–774, available from: PM:16226956

Balcombe J (2004) Medical training using simulation: toward fewer animals and safer patients. Altern Lab Anim 32(Suppl 1B):553–560, available from: PM:23581135

Bell RH Jr (2004) Alternative training models for surgical residency. Surg Clin North Am 84(6):1699–1711, xii available from: PM:15501282

Bholat OS, Haluck RS, Murray WB, Gorman PJ, Krummel TM (1999) Tactile feedback is present during minimally invasive surgery. J Am Coll Surg 189(4):349–355, available from: PM:10509459

Biggs J (2003) Constructing learning by aligning teaching: constructive alignment. In: Biggs J (ed) Teaching for quality learning at university, 2nd edn. Open University Press, Berkshire, pp 11–33

Birkhahn RH, Jauch E, Kramer DA, Nowak RM, Raja AS, Summers RL, Weber JE, Diercks DB (2009) A review of the federal guidelines that inform and influence relationships between physicians and industry. Acad Emerg Med 16(8):776–781, available from: PM:19594459

Bloom BS, Engelhart MD, Furst EJ, Hill WH, Kratwohl DR (1956) Taxonomy of educational objectives, the classification of educational goals – Handboek I: cognitive domain. McKay, New York

Boyle E, Al-Akash M, Gallagher AG, Traynor O, Hill AD, Neary PC (2011) Optimising surgical training: use of feedback to reduce errors during a simulated surgical procedure. Postgrad Med J 87(1030):524–528, available from: PM:21642446

Braun DA, Aertsen A, Wolpert DM, Mehring C (2009) Motor task variation induces structural learning. Curr Biol 19(4):352–357, available from: PM:19217296

Braun DA, Mehring C, Wolpert DM (2010) Structure learning in action. Behav Brain Res 206(2):157–165, available from: PM:19720086

Brown J, Collins A, Duguid P (1989) Situated cognition and the culture of learning. Educ Res 18(1):32–42

Butler A, Olson T, Koehler R, Nicandri G (2013) Do the skills acquired by novice surgeons using anatomic dry models transfer effectively to the task of diagnostic knee arthroscopy performed on cadaveric specimens? J Bone Joint Surg Am 95(3):e15–e18, available from: PM:23380705

Castricini R, De BM, Orlando N, Rocchi M, Zini R, Pirani P (2013) Arthroscopic Latarjet procedure: analysis of the learning curve. Musculoskelet Surg 97(Suppl 1):93–98, available from: PM:23588833

Chami G, Ward JW, Phillips R, Sherman KP (2008) Haptic feedback can provide an objective assessment of arthroscopic skills. Clin Orthop Relat Res 466(4):963–968, available from: PM:18213507

Clark R, Mayer R (2011) E-learning and the science of instruction: proven guidelines for consumers and designers of multimedia learning, 3rd edn. John Wiley & Sons, Pfeiffer.

Commision of the European Communities (2006) Adult learning: It is never too late to learn. 30-5-2014. Ref Type: Online Source. http://eur-lex.europa.eu/legal-content/EN/ALL/?uri=CELEX:52006DC0614

Committee on Ethics and Standards and the Board of Directors of the Arthroscopy Association of North America (2008) Suggested guidelines for the practice of arthroscopic surgery. Arthroscopy 24(6):A30, available from: PM:18536081

Cullen KA, Hall MJ, Golosinskiy A (2009) Ambulatory surgery in the United States, 2006. Natl Health Stat Report (11):1–25 available from: PM:19294964

Dankelman J, Chmarra MK, Verdaasdonk EG, Stassen LP, Grimbergen CA (2005) Fundamental aspects of learning minimally invasive surgical skills. Minim Invasive Ther Allied Technol 14(4):247–256, available from: PM:16754171

Dave RH (1970) Psychomotor levels. In: Armstrong RJ (ed) Developing and writing behavioral objectives. Educational Innovators Press, Tucson

Davidson PR, Wolpert DM (2003) Motor learning and prediction in a variable environment. Curr Opin Neurobiol 13(2):232–237, available from: PM:12744979

Dawson SL, Kaufman JA (1998) The imperative for medical simulation. Proc IEEE 86(3):479–483, available from: ISI:000072454200003

Endsley MR (1995) Toward a theory of situation awareness in dynamic-systems. Hum Factors 37(1):32–64, available from: ISI:A1995RL73500004

Engineers AASoM (2000) The Link Flight Trainer: a historical mechanical engineering landmark. 31-1-2014. Ref Type: Online Source. https://www.asme.org/getmedia/d75b81fd-83e8-4458-aba7-166a87d35811/210-Link-C-3-Flight-Trainer.aspx

Escoto A, Le BF, Trejos AL, Naish MD, Patel RV, Lebel ME (2013) A knee arthroscopy simulator: design and validation. Conf Proc IEEE Eng Med Biol Soc 2013:5715–5718, available from: PM:24111035

Eversbusch A, Grantcharov TP (2004) Learning curves and impact of psychomotor training on performance in simulated colonoscopy: a randomized trial using a virtual reality endoscopy trainer. Surg Endosc 18(10):1514–1518, available from: PM:15791380

Fitts PM, Posner MI (1967) Human performance. Brooks/Cole, Belmont

Flanagan JR, Vetter P, Johansson RS, Wolpert DM (2003) Prediction precedes control in motor learning. Curr Biol 13(2):146–150, available from: PM:12546789

France DJ, Leming-Lee S, Jackson T, Feistritzer NR, Higgins MS (2008) An observational analysis of surgical team compliance with perioperative safety practices after crew resource management training. Am J Surg 195(4):546–553, available from: PM:18304501

Frank RM, Erickson B, Frank JM, Bush-Joseph CA, Bach BR Jr, Cole BJ, Romeo AA, Provencher MT, Verma NN (2014) Utility of modern arthroscopic simulator training models. Arthroscopy 30(1):121–133, available from: PM:24290789

Gagne R (1965) The conditions of learning. Holt, Rinehart and Winston. Inc, New York

Gallagher AG, Ritter EM, Lederman AB, McClusky DA III, Smith CD (2005) Video-assisted surgery represents more than a loss of three-dimensional vision. Am J Surg 189(1):76–80, available from: PM:15701497

Gallagher AG, Leonard G, Traynor OJ (2009) Role and feasibility of psychomotor and dexterity testing in selection for surgical training. ANZ J Surg 79(3):108–113, available from: PM:19317772

Gallagher AG, Jordan-Black JA, O'Sullivan GC (2012) Prospective, randomized assessment of the acquisition, maintenance, and loss of laparoscopic skills. Ann Surg 256(2):387–393, available from: PM:22580935

Gardner H (2011) Frames of mind: the theory of multiple intelligences, 3rd edn. Basic Books, New York

Garrett WE Jr, Swiontkowski MF, Weinstein JN, Callaghan J, Rosier RN, Berry DJ, Harrast J, Derosa GP (2006) American Board of Orthopaedic Surgery Practice of the Orthopaedic Surgeon: Part-II, certification examination case mix. J Bone Joint Surg Am 88(3):660–667, available from: PM:16510834

Gawande AA, Zinner MJ, Studdert DM, Brennan TA (2003) Analysis of errors reported by surgeons at three teaching hospitals. Surgery 133(6):614–621, available from: PM:12796727

Georgoulis A, Randelli P (2011) Education in arthroscopy, sports medicine and knee surgery. Knee Surg Sports Traumatol Arthrosc 19(8):1231–1232, available from: PM:21630049

Gomoll AH, Pappas G, Forsythe B, Warner JJ (2008) Individual skill progression on a virtual reality simulator for shoulder arthroscopy: a 3-year follow-up study. Am J Sports Med 36(6):1139–1142, available from: PM:18326032

Grechenig W, Fellinger M, Fankhauser F, Weiglein AH (1999) The Graz learning and training model for arthroscopic surgery. Surg Radiol Anat 21(5):347–350, available from: PM:10635100

Grogan EL, Stiles RA, France DJ, Speroff T, Morris JA Jr, Nixon B, Gaffney FA, Seddon R, Pinson CW (2004) The impact of aviation-based teamwork training on the attitudes of health-care professionals. J Am Coll Surg 199(6):843–848, available from: PM:15555963

Hall MP, Kaplan KM, Gorczynski CT, Zuckerman JD, Rosen JE (2010) Assessment of arthroscopic training in U.S. orthopedic surgery residency programs–a resident self-assessment. Bull NYU Hosp Jt Dis 68(1):5–10, available from: PM:20345354

Hanna GB, Shimi SM, Cuschieri A (1998) Randomised study of influence of two-dimensional versus three-dimensional imaging on performance of laparoscopic cholecystectomy. Lancet 351(9098):248–251, available from: PM:9457094

Harewood GC, Murray F, Winder S, Patchett S (2008) Evaluation of formal feedback on endoscopic competence among trainees: the EFFECT trial. Ir J Med Sci 177(3):253–256, available from: PM:18584274

Haward D (1910) The Sanders teacher. Flight 2(50): 1006–1007

Hawes R, Lehman GA, Hast J, O'Connor KW, Crabb DW, Lui A, Christiansen PA (1986) Training resident physicians in fiberoptic sigmoidoscopy. How many supervised examinations are required to achieve competence? Am J Med 80(3):465–470, available from: PM:3953621

Henn RF III, Shah N, Warner JJ, Gomoll AH (2013) Shoulder arthroscopy simulator training improves shoulder arthroscopy performance in a cadaveric model. Arthroscopy 29(6):982–985, available from: PM:23591380

Hmelo-Silver CE (2004) Problem-based learning: what and how do students learn? Edu Psychol Rev 16(3):235–266, available from: ISI:000222473700003

Hodgins JL, Veillette C (2013) Arthroscopic proficiency: methods in evaluating competency. BMC Med Educ 13:61, available from: PM:23631421

Hogan MP, Pace DE, Hapgood J, Boone DC (2006) Use of human patient simulation and the situation awareness global assessment technique in practical trauma skills assessment. J Trauma 61(5):1047–1052, available from: PM:17099507

Hoppe DJ, de SD, Simunovic N, Bhandari M, Safran MR, Larson CM, Ayeni OR (2014) The learning curve for hip arthroscopy: a systematic review. Arthroscopy 30:389–397, available from: PM:24461140

Horeman T, Rodrigues SP, Jansen FW, Dankelman J, van den Dobbelsteen JJ (2010) Force measurement platform for training and assessment of laparoscopic skills. Surg Endosc 24(12):3102–3108, available from: PM:20464416

Horeman T, Rodrigues SP, van den Dobbelsteen JJ, Jansen FW, Dankelman J (2012) Visual force feedback in laparoscopic training. Surg Endosc 26(1):242–248, available from: PM:21858573

Horton W (2011) E-learning by design, 2nd edn. Wiley & Sons, Pfeiffer.

Howells NR, Brinsden MD, Gill RS, Carr AJ, Rees JL (2008a) Motion analysis: a validated method for showing skill levels in arthroscopy. Arthroscopy 24(3):335–342, available from: PM:18308187

Howells NR, Gill HS, Carr AJ, Price AJ, Rees JL (2008b) Transferring simulated arthroscopic skills to the operating theatre: a randomised blinded study. J Bone Joint Surg Br 90(4):494–499, available from: PM:18378926

Howells NR, Auplish S, Hand GC, Gill HS, Carr AJ, Rees JL (2009) Retention of arthroscopic shoulder skills learned with use of a simulator. Demonstration of a learning curve and loss of performance level after a time delay. J Bone Joint Surg Am 91(5):1207–1213, available from: PM:19411470

Hui Y, Safir O, Dubrowski A, Carnahan H (2013) What skills should simulation training in arthroscopy teach residents? A focus on resident input. Int J Comput Assist Radiol Surg 8:945–953, available from: PM:23535939

Hurmusiadis V, Rhode K, Schaeffter T, Sherman K (2011) Virtual arthroscopy trainer for minimally invasive surgery. Stud Health Technol Inform 163:236–238, available from: PM:21335795

Jonassen D (1999) Designing constructivist learning environments. Instr Des Theor Models New Paradigm Instr Theory 2:215–239

Karahan M, Unalan PC, Bozkurt S, Odabas I, Akgun U, Cifcili S, Lobenhoffer P, Aydin AT (2009) Correlation of basic motor skills with arthroscopic experience. Acta Orthop Traumatol Turc 43(1):49–53, available from: PM:19293616

Kaufman HH, Wiegand RL, Tunick RH (1987) Teaching surgeons to operate–principles of psychomotor skills training. Acta Neurochir (Wien) 87(1–2):1–7, available from: PM:3314366

Kawato M (1999) Internal models for motor control and trajectory planning. Curr Opin Neurobiol 9(6):718–727, available from: PM:10607637

Kim RH, Gilbert T, Ristig K, Chu QD (2013) Surgical resident learning styles: faculty and resident accuracy at identification of preferences and impact on ABSITE scores. J Surg Res 184(1):31–36, available from: PM:23706561

Kissin EY, Schiller AM, Gelbard RB, Anderson JJ, Falanga V, Simms RW, Korn JH, Merkel PA (2006) Durometry for the assessment of skin disease in systemic sclerosis. Arthritis Rheum 55(4):603–609, available from: PM:16874783

Kitson J, Blake SM (2006) A model for developing psychomotor skills in arthroscopic knot tying. Ann R Coll Surg Engl 88(5):501–502, available from: PM:17009424

Koehler RJ, Nicandri GT (2013) Using the arthroscopic surgery skill evaluation tool as a pass-fail examination. J Bone Joint Surg Am 95(23):e1871–e1876, available from: PM:24306710

Kohn L, Corrigan J, Donaldson M (2000) To err is human: building a safer health system. National Academy Press, Washington DC

Kording KP, Wolpert DM (2004) Bayesian integration in sensorimotor learning. Nature 427(6971):244–247, available from: PM:14724638

Leonard M, Kennedy J, Kiely P, Murphy P (2007) Knee arthroscopy: how much training is necessary? A cross-sectional study. Eur J Orthop Surg Traumatol 17:359–362

Lingard L, Espin S, Whyte S, Regehr G, Baker GR, Reznick R, Bohnen J, Orser B, Doran D, Grober E (2004) Communication failures in the operating room: an observational classification of recurrent types and effects. Qual Saf Health Care 13(5):330–334, available from: PM:15465935

Madan SS, Pai DR (2014) Role of simulation in arthroscopy training. Simul Healthc 9(2):127–135, available from: PM:24096921

Mattos e Dinato MC, Freitas MF, Iutaka AS (2010) A porcine model for arthroscopy. Foot Ankle Int 31(2):179–181, available from: PM:20132758

Megali G, Tonet O, Dario P, Vascellari A, Marcacci M (2005) Computer-assisted training system for knee arthroscopy. Int J Med Robot 1(3):57–66, available from: PM:17518391

Merriam S, Caffarella R, Baumgartner L (2012) Learning in adulthood: a comprehensive guide. John Wiley & Sons, New York

Merrienboer J, Clark S, Croock M (2002) Blueprints for complex learning: the 4C/ID-model. Educ Tech Res Develop 50:39–64

Meyer RD, Tamarapalli JR, Lemons JE (1993) Arthroscopy training using a "black box" technique. Arthroscopy 9(3):338–340, available from: PM:8323624

Miller WE (1985) Learning arthroscopy. South Med J 78(8):935–937, available from: PM:4023785

Modi CS, Morris G, Mukherjee R (2010) Computer-simulation training for knee and shoulder arthroscopic surgery. Arthroscopy 26(6):832–840, available from: PM:20511043

Morris AH, Jennings JE, Stone RG, Katz JA, Garroway RY, Hendler RC (1993) Guidelines for privileges in arthroscopic surgery. Arthroscopy 9(1):125–127, available from: PM:8442822

Neequaye SK, Aggarwal R, Brightwell R, Van Herzeele I, Darzi A, Cheshire NJ (2007) Identification of skills common to renal and iliac endovascular procedures performed on a virtual reality simulator. Eur J Vasc Endovasc Surg 33(5):525–532, available from: PM:17291792

Neily J, Mills PD, Young-Xu Y, Carney BT, West P, Berger DH, Mazzia LM, Paull DE, Bagian JP (2010) Association between implementation of a medical team training program and surgical mortality. JAMA 304(15):1693–1700, available from: PM:20959579

Neiman Z (1989) Teaching specific motor skills for conducting to young music students. Percept Mot Skills 68(3 Pt 1):847–858, available from: PM:2748301

O'Connor A, Schwaitzberg SD, Cao CG (2008) How much feedback is necessary for learning to suture? Surg Endosc 22(7):1614–1619, available from: PM:17973165

O'Neill PJ, Cosgarea AJ, Freedman JA, Queale WS, McFarland EG (2002) Arthroscopic proficiency: a survey of orthopaedic sports medicine fellowship directors and orthopaedic surgery department chairs. Arthroscopy 18(7):795–800, available from: PM:12209439

Obdeijn MC, Bavinck N, Mathoulin C, van der Horst CM, Schijven MP, Tuijthof GJ (2013) Education in wrist arthroscopy: past, present and future. Knee Surg Sports Traumatol Arthrosc. available from: PM:23835770

Obdeijn MC, Alewijnse JV, Mathoulin C, Liverneaux P, Tuijthof GJ, Schijven MP (2014) Development and validation of a computer-based learning module for wrist arthroscopy. Chir Main 33:100–105, available from: PM:24560535

Omrod J, Davis K (2004) Human learning. Merrill, London

Oxford English Dictionary. Oxford University Press. http://www.oed.com/. Acessed 15 Jan 2014

Paige JT, Kozmenko V, Yang T, Paragi GR, Hilton CW, Cohn I Jr, Chauvin SW (2009) High-fidelity, simulation-based, interdisciplinary operating room team training at the point of care. Surgery 145(2):138–146, available from: PM:19167968

Paris S, Winograd P (1990) How metacognition can promote academic learning and instruction. Dimens Think Cogn Instr 1:15–51

Patel D, Guhl JF (1983) The use of bovine knees in operative arthroscopy. Orthopedics 6(9):1119–1124, available from: PM:24822909

Patel VM, Warren O, Humphris P, Ahmed K, Ashrafian H, Rao C, Athanasiou T, Darzi A (2010) What does leadership in surgery entail? ANZ J Surg 80(12):876–883, available from: PM:21114726

Patil V, Odak S, Chian V, Chougle A (2009) Use of webcam as arthroscopic training model for junior surgical trainees. Ann R Coll Surg Engl 91(2):161–162, available from: PM:19579297

Pedowitz RA, Esch J, Snyder S (2002) Evaluation of a virtual reality simulator for arthroscopy skills development. Arthroscopy 18(6):E29, available from: PM:12098111

Poehling GG, Lubowitz JH, Brand R, Buckwalter JA, Wright TM, Canale ST, Cooney WP III, D'Ambrosia R, Frassica FJ, Grana WA, Heckman JD, Hensinger RN, Thompson GH, Koman LA, McCann PD, Thordarson D (2008) Patient care, professionalism, and relations with industry. Arthroscopy 24(1):4–6, available from: PM:18182194

Pories W (1999) Some reflections on Halsted and residency training. Curr Surg 56(1–2):1

Rosen KR (2008) The history of medical simulation. J Crit Care 23(2):157–166, available from: PM:18538206

Rovai AP, Wighting MJ, Baker JD, Grooms LD (2009) Development of an instrument to measure perceived cognitive, affective, and psychomotor learning in traditional and virtual classroom higher education settings. Internet Higher Educ 12(1):7–13, available from: ISI:000264833900002

Safir O, Dubrowski A, Mirsky L, Lin C, Backstein D, Carnahan A (2008) What skills should simulation training in arthroscopy teach residents? Int J Comput Assist Radiol Surg 3(5):433–437

Satava RM (1993) Virtual reality surgical simulator. The first steps. Surg Endosc 7(3):203–205, available from: PM:8503081

Schaafsma BE, Hiemstra E, Dankelman J, Jansen FW (2009) Feedback in laparoscopic skills acquisition: an observational study during a basic skills training course. Gynecol Surg 6(4):339–343, available from: PM:20234844

Sealy W (1999) Halsted is dead: time for change in graduate surgical education. Curr Surg 56(1–2):34–38

Seidler RD (2007) Older adults can learn to learn new motor skills. Behav Brain Res 183(1):118–122, available from: PM:17602760

Sexton JB, Thomas EJ, Helmreich RL (2000) Error, stress, and teamwork in medicine and aviation: cross sectional surveys. BMJ 320(7237):745–749, available from: PM:10720356

Shadmehr R, Smith MA, Krakauer JW (2010) Error correction, sensory prediction, and adaptation in motor control. Annu Rev Neurosci 33:89–108, available from: PM:20367317

Shearer CB (1998) MIDAS: Multiple Intelligences Developmental Assessment Scales, Adult Version. Corwin, USA

Sherman KP, Ward JW, Wills DP, Sherman VJ, Mohsen AM (2001) Surgical trainee assessment using a VE knee arthroscopy training system (VE-KATS): experimental results. Stud Health Technol Inform 81:465–470, available from: PM:11317792

Simpson EJ (1972) The classification of educational objectives in the psychomotor domain. Gryphon House, Washington, DC

Slade Shantz JA, Leiter JR, Collins JB, MacDonald PB (2013) Validation of a global assessment of arthroscopic skills in a cadaveric knee model. Arthroscopy 29(1):106–112, available from: PM:23177383

Slade Shantz JA, Leiter JR, Gottschalk T, MacDonald PB (2014) The internal validity of arthroscopic simulators and their effectiveness in arthroscopic education. Knee Surg Sports Traumatol Arthrosc 22(1):33–40, available from: PM:23052120

Smeets JB, van den Dobbelsteen JJ, de Grave DD, van Beers RJ, Brenner E (2006) Sensory integration does not lead to sensory calibration. Proc Natl Acad Sci U S A 103(49):18781–18786, available from: PM:17130453

Splawski R (2011) Animal model of humeral joint for shoulder arthroscopy training. Chir Narzadow Ruchu Ortop Pol 76(6):324–326, available from: PM:22708318

Straub RO, Terrace HS (1981) Generalization of serial-learning in the pigeon. Anim Learn Behav 9(4):454–468, available from: ISI:A1981MZ83400003

Strom P, Kjellin A, Hedman L, Wredmark T, Fellander-Tsai L (2004) Training in tasks with different visual-spatial components does not improve virtual arthroscopy performance. Surg Endosc 18(1):115–120, available from: PM:14625735

Suksudaj N, Townsend GC, Kaidonis J, Lekkas D, Winning TA (2012) Acquiring psychomotor skills in operative dentistry: do innate ability and motivation matter? Eur J Dent Educ 16(1):e187–e194, available from: PM:22251344

Sulzenbruck S, Heuer H (2012) Enhanced mechanical transparency during practice impedes open-loop control of a complex tool. Exp Brain Res 218(2):283–294, available from: PM:22278111

Tashiro Y, Miura H, Nakanishi Y, Okazaki K, Iwamoto Y (2009) Evaluation of skills in arthroscopic training based on trajectory and force data. Clin Orthop Relat Res 467(2):546–552, available from: PM:18791774

Thomas W (2008) The making of a surgeon. Surgery (Oxford) 26(10):400–402

Tokuhama-Espinosa T (2010) Mind, brain, and education science: a comprehensive guide to the new brain-based teaching, 1st edn. W.W. Norton & Company Inc, New York

Triano JJ, Scaringe J, Bougie J, Rogers C (2006) Effects of visual feedback on manipulation performance and patient ratings. J Manipulative Physiol Ther 29(5):378–385, available from: PM:16762666

Tuijthof G, de Wit M, Horeman T, Kerkhoffs G. Evaluation of PASSPORT v2, 22th Annual meeting of the Dutch Arthroscopy Association, ed., Den Bosch

Tuijthof GJM, Horeman T (2011) Training facility, surgical instruments and artificial knee with an upper limb and a lower limb for simulation and training of arthroscopic surgical techniques. Patent N2006846

Tuijthof GJ, van Sterkenburg MN, Sierevelt IN, Van OJ, van Dijk CN, Kerkhoffs GM (2010) First validation of the PASSPORT training environment for arthroscopic skills. Knee Surg Sports Traumatol Arthrosc 18(2):218–224, available from: PM:19629441

Tuijthof GJ, Visser P, Sierevelt IN, van Dijk CN, Kerkhoffs GM (2011) Does perception of usefulness of arthroscopic simulators differ with levels of experience? Clin Orthop Relat Res 469:1701–1708, available from: PM:21290203

Unalan PC, Akan K, Orhun H, Akgun U, Poyanli O, Baykan A, Yavuz Y, Beyzadeoglu T, Nuran R, Kocaoglu B, Topsakal N, Akman M, Karahan M (2010) A basic arthroscopy course based on motor skill training. Knee Surg Sports Traumatol Arthrosc 18(10):1395–1399, available from: PM:20012013

Undre S, Koutantji M, Sevdalis N, Gautama S, Selvapatt N, Williams S, Sains P, McCulloch P, Darzi A, Vincent C (2007) Multidisciplinary crisis simulations: the way forward for training surgical teams. World J Surg 31(9):1843–1853, available from: PM:17610109

van Beers RJ (2009) Motor learning is optimally tuned to the properties of motor noise. Neuron 63(3):406–417, available from: PM:19679079

Verdaasdonk EG, Stassen LP, Schijven MP, Dankelman J (2007) Construct validity and assessment of the learning curve for the SIMENDO endoscopic simulator. Surg Endosc 21(8):1406–1412, available from: PM:17653815

Vitale MA, Kleweno CP, Jacir AM, Levine WN, Bigliani LU, Ahmad CS (2007) Training resources in arthroscopic rotator cuff repair. J Bone Joint Surg Am 89(6):1393–1398, available from: PM:17545443

Voto SJ, Clark RN, Zuelzer WA (1988) Arthroscopic training using pig knee joints. Clin Orthop Relat Res 226:134–137, available from: PM:3335089

Wanzel KR, Ward M, Reznick RK (2002) Teaching the surgical craft: from selection to certification. Curr Probl Surg 39(6):573–659, available from: PM:12037512

Wentink M, Breedveld P, Stassen LP, Oei IH, Wieringa PA (2002) A clearly visible endoscopic instrument shaft on the monitor facilitates hand-eye coordination. Surg Endosc 16(11):1533–1537, available from: PM:12072991

Windsor JA, Diener S, Zoha F (2008) Learning style and laparoscopic experience in psychomotor skill performance using a virtual reality surgical simulator. Am J Surg 195(6):837–842, available from: PM:18417084

Wirth K, Malone B, Barrera K, Widmann WD, Turner C, Sanni A (2014) Is there a place for medical students as teachers in the education of junior residents? Am J Surg 207(2):271–274, available from: PM:24468027

Wolf BR, Britton CL (2013) How orthopaedic residents perceive educational resources. Iowa Orthop J 33:185–190, available from: PM:24027481

Wolpert DM, Ghahramani Z (2000) Computational principles of movement neuroscience. Nat Neurosci 3(Suppl):1212–1217, available from: PM:11127840

Wolpert DM, Miall RC (1996) Forward models for physiological motor control. Neural Netw 9(8):1265–1279, available from: PM:12662535

Woolley NN, Jarvis Y (2007) Situated cognition and cognitive apprenticeship: a model for teaching and learning clinical skills in a technologically rich and authentic learning environment. Nurse Educ Today 27(1):73–79, available from: PM:16624452

Enabling Lifelong Learning and Team Skills to Support Arthroscopic Performance

4

Jan Maarten Luursema, Kevin Sherman, and Jenny Dankelman

Now, here, you see, it takes all the running you can do, to keep in the same place – The Red Queen

Take-Home Messages

- The integration of medical knowledge, team skills and psychomotor skills is a prerequisite for high-quality operating room performance.
- Arthroscopic surgeons need to possess knowledge acquisition skills to support lifelong learning.
- Well-designed and implemented digital learning tools can support lifelong arthroscopy learning.
- Cognitive apprenticeship offers a holistic training approach well suited to prepare the resident for continued learning in the operating room

J.M. Luursema (✉)
Department of Surgery, RadboudUMC,
Nijmegen, The Netherlands
e-mail: Jan-maarten.Luursema@radboudumc.nl

K. Sherman, MD
Department of Orthopedics, Castle Hill Hospital,
Cottingham, East Yorkshire, UK
e-mail: kp_sherman@hotmail.com

J. Dankelman
Department of Biomechanical Engineering,
Delft University of Technology, Delft, The Netherlands
e-mail: J.Dankelman@tudelft.nl

4.1 Definitions

Learning We offer the following definition of learning: an increase in behavioural repertoire or knowledge, resulting from personal experience or transmission of knowledge.

Education When people learn in conditions that are created to optimise and to standardise learning, this is called education.

Metacognition is the ability to recognise one's need for additional learning and training, to seek out opportunities for such learning and to critically reflect on one's progress towards self-set learning goals (Paris and Winograd 1990).

Crew resource management entails a set of training procedures for use in environments where human error can have devastating effects.

4.2 Introduction

As outlined in previous chapters, arthroscopic skills training is increasingly moving away from the operating room, due to patient safety concerns, the need to increase training efficiency and the need to limit costs (Dawson and Kaufman 1998). However, psychomotor arthroscopic skills need to be complemented with team skills and a relevant body of arthroscopic knowledge, before the resident can start integrating knowledge *and* skills in the operating room (Georgoulis and Randelli 2011).

M. Karahan et al. (eds.), *Effective Training of Arthroscopic Skills*,
DOI 10.1007/978-3-662-44943-1_4, © ESSKA 2015

In this chapter, we will first discuss learning and the requirements for designing a successful knowledge course based on state-of-the-art digital technology. Subsequently, we will discuss team skills such as crew resource management (CRM), communication skills, leadership and situation awareness and how to train such skills using simulation.

4.2.1 Learning and Education

Early paradigms in education emphasised producing desired behaviour by reward and punishment or viewed people as analytical, information processing entities that can be trained to apply conditional rules to situations (Omrod and Davis 2004). Recognition that people are individual, intentional agents (Jonassen 1999), the currently predominant educational paradigm of constructivism has spawned a number of approaches that build on and go beyond these earlier paradigms.

Constructivism is the umbrella term that covers most contemporary approaches to education and educational research. It emphasises learning in a 'realistic' environment, the need to engage trainee motivation and the student's capacity to self-direct learning. Constructivist approaches relevant to the aims of this chapter are problem-based learning (Hmelo-Silver 2004), lifelong learning (Merriam et al. 2012) and cognitive apprenticeship (Brown et al. 1989).

4.2.2 Problem-Based Learning

Classical classroom education has a tendency to create 'hurdlers', students for whom passing a series of pass or fail tests is driving learning (Amrein and Berliner 2002). There is a discrepancy between such short-term goals and the patient-centred goals we want our professionals to adopt. Problem-based learning aims to alleviate this problem by providing trainees with learning materials based on real-world cases (Omrod and Davis 2004). In this way, knowledge can be gained in a patient-based learning framework. Students work in groups and have to develop both problem-solving strategies and content

knowledge. The educator takes on the role of facilitator in this approach. Rather than training courses culminating in pieces of paper with grades on them, students develop a portfolio to document their experience and skills.

4.2.3 Metacognition for Lifelong Learning

In arthroscopy as in most fields of medicine, knowledge, technology and procedures are changing with increasing speed. The modern professional cannot expect to learn once and perform ever after. Arthroscopic surgeons need to learn how to be lifelong trainees in order to stay up to date and remain competitive in an increasingly consumer-driven marketplace. Implementing problem-based learning early in the curriculum can ease the transition from learning in an educational setting to lifelong learning.

After initial knowledge is gained, modern professionals need to make the transition to becoming lifelong learners. This is contingent upon the trainee developing metacognition (Paris and Winograd 1990). Lifelong learning is recognised by amongst others the European Union as a prime directive in maintaining a flexible workforce (Commission of the European Communities 2007). It is also part of the suggested guidelines for the practice of arthroscopic surgery as outlined by the Committee on Ethics and Standards and the Board of Directors of the Arthroscopy Association of North America (2008).

Simulation training is well suited to help develop metacognition, as it isolates critical aspects of professional practice and provides the trainee with objective and quantified feedback (Chaps. 6, 7, 9, and 11). This helps students to keep track of their progress towards learning and training goals and stimulates critical reflection (Paris and Winograd 1990). However, lifelong learning goes beyond training practical skills and needs to include knowledge goals to make sure practical skills are applied appropriately. This is a broad area, which ranges from the statistical knowledge necessary to identify best treatment options for a specific patient's pathology (evidence-based medicine) to refresher/advanced courses in anatomy, pathology, arthroscopy, etc. E-learning can be used to provide the lifelong learner with this extra knowledge on an as-needed, just-in-time basis and can be used for assessment as well.

4.3 E-Learning Design

The independence digital media allows from the classroom to makes it easy and attractive to implement problem-based learning and life-long lifelong learning strategies in the workplace (Obdeijn et al. 2014). The trainee is flexible in selecting time and place to engage in learning on an as-needed basis. Formative assessment (intended to provide feedback to the trainee) is easily implemented in such environments. Summative assessment (is the trainee well enough equipped to practise this or that procedure) is harder to implement, given the lack of control this flexibility brings along.

Afforded by the everyday use of networked computers, the flexibility, efficiency and effectiveness of e-learning have caused this to be a booming field since the late 1990s. However, developing e-learning is an involved process that includes developing learning goals, training course design, assessment, usability testing and creating appropriate multimedia illustrations. A full treatment of this field is outside the scope of this chapter, and the reader is referred to standard works on this subject, such as Clark and Mayer (2011) and Horton (2011). In the following section, nine instructional design principles are discussed to keep in mind when developing e-learning and training programmes in general.

4.3.1 Gagne's Instructional Design Principles

Gagne's work was very important for the development of instructions in the military. For example, during World War II, many technicians and pilots needed training of highly complex tasks. By implementing a systematic approach to training, *farm boys transformed into airplane mechanics in 30 days instead of 2 years*. Gagne identified

1. Gaining attention of the trainee. This is, for example, done by a demonstration of something that can go wrong in the actual worlds: This is a problem in the real operating room; therefore, training outside the operating room is necessary.
2. Inform the trainee about the objectives of the course/lesson. These objectives will help the trainee to organise their thoughts around what they are about to see, hear and/or do. Schaafsma and coworkers (2009) investigated what has been learned after a basic laparoscopic skill training and concluded that it is crucial that training objectives are clear prior to a course for both the expert and the trainee; otherwise, some important skill or knowledge might not be acquired.
3. Stimulating recalling of prior knowledge. This can make trainees build on their personal experience and previous knowledge and skills.
4. Present the material in an organised and meaningful way and divide it into familiar manageable units.
5. Provide guidance for learning. This can be giving by examples, non-examples, case studies, graphical representations, mnemonics and analogies.
6. Elicit performance. Allow the trainee to do something with the newly acquired behaviour, skills or knowledge. Repetition increases the likelihood of retention.
7. Provide specific and immediate feedback. Studies carried out in (simulated) operative settings suggested indeed that knowledge on their performance given in a systematic manner enhances training (Harewood et al. 2008; O'Connor et al. 2008).
8. Assess performance to determine if the lesson has been learned.
9. Enhance retention and transfer. Inform the trainee about similar problem situations, provide additional practice, put the trainee in a transfer situation and review the lesson (Gagne 1965).

nine events that activate processes needed for effective learning (Gagne 1965):

4.3.2 Examples of E-Learning Courses in Arthroscopy

Simulation training for surgical procedures is increasingly seen as an essential component of the curriculum. In the UK, compulsory simulation training is for the first time being introduced into the curriculum by the regulator, the General Medical Council. It is almost certain that this trend will continue.

Any practical procedure can be broken down into its component parts using the technique of hierarchical task analysis. Those components that cause difficulty for trainees can be identified. The arthroscopic skills involved can be divided into *cognitive* and *haptic*. The cognitive aspects could be trained with an online simulator, where the programme is held on a central server and where the simulator addresses those aspects of a surgical task that do not require a complex end user controller. The concept of a *cognitive trainer* for arthroscopy of the knee was explored by the Royal College of Surgeons of England in collaboration with Primal Pictures. This resulted in the pilot VATMAS simulator, which was built on earlier work on the VE-KATS simulator (Fig. 4.1) (Sherman et al. 2001). This tutorial-based simulator uses a simple and cheap interface to address the cognitive *non-haptic* components of arthroscopic knee surgery (Hurmusiadis et al. 2011).

An *overview* can be provided if the trainee became disorientated (Fig. 4.1). Additionally, the VATMAS simulator can take the trainee through a series of tutorials, whilst providing automated feedback based on time, accuracy and efficiency. From any point, images or videos from real arthroscopies can be called up. Finally, the arthroscope and probe can be independently manipulated with indication of contact with hard and soft surfaces.

Another example of development of an e-learning module was recently presented by Obeijn and coworkers who focused on wrist arthroscopy (Obdeijn et al. 2014). The need for such a module

was assessed by questioning the members of the European Wrist Arthroscopy Society (EWAS). The e-learning module consisted of seven topics important for wrist arthroscopy: indications, patient positioning, traction, instruments, portals, entry procedure and radio-carpal anatomy. The e-learning module did not show learning enhancement in a randomised controlled trial with 28 medical students. However, the participants did find the module more pleasant to use, and its content is fully supported by a panel of experts. This module is a typical example of a flexible easy to engage and delivered as needed to support lifelong learning.

4.4 Team Skills

Besides psychomotor skills, up-to-date knowledge and knowledge acquisition skills, team skills are the third essential component for the arthroscopic surgeon. Since the ground-breaking report *To Err Is Human* (Kohn et al. 2000), we know that many medical errors are not errors of judgement or skill, but instead are caused by ineffective team cooperation and communication. Crew resource management (CRM) skills, which include communication skills, leadership skills and situation awareness, need to be trained to ensure safety in the operating room. How these skills after initial training can be further monitored in the operating room is covered in Chap. 14. We will continue with a discussion of CRM, communication, leadership and situation awareness.

4.4.1 Crew Resource Management

CRM is an approach borrowed from the airline industry but increasingly applied to the medical domain. Crew resource management entails a set of training procedures for use in environments where human error can have devastating effects. It encompasses a wide range of knowledge, skills and attitudes including interpersonal communications, situational awareness, problem-solving, decision-making, leadership and teamwork.

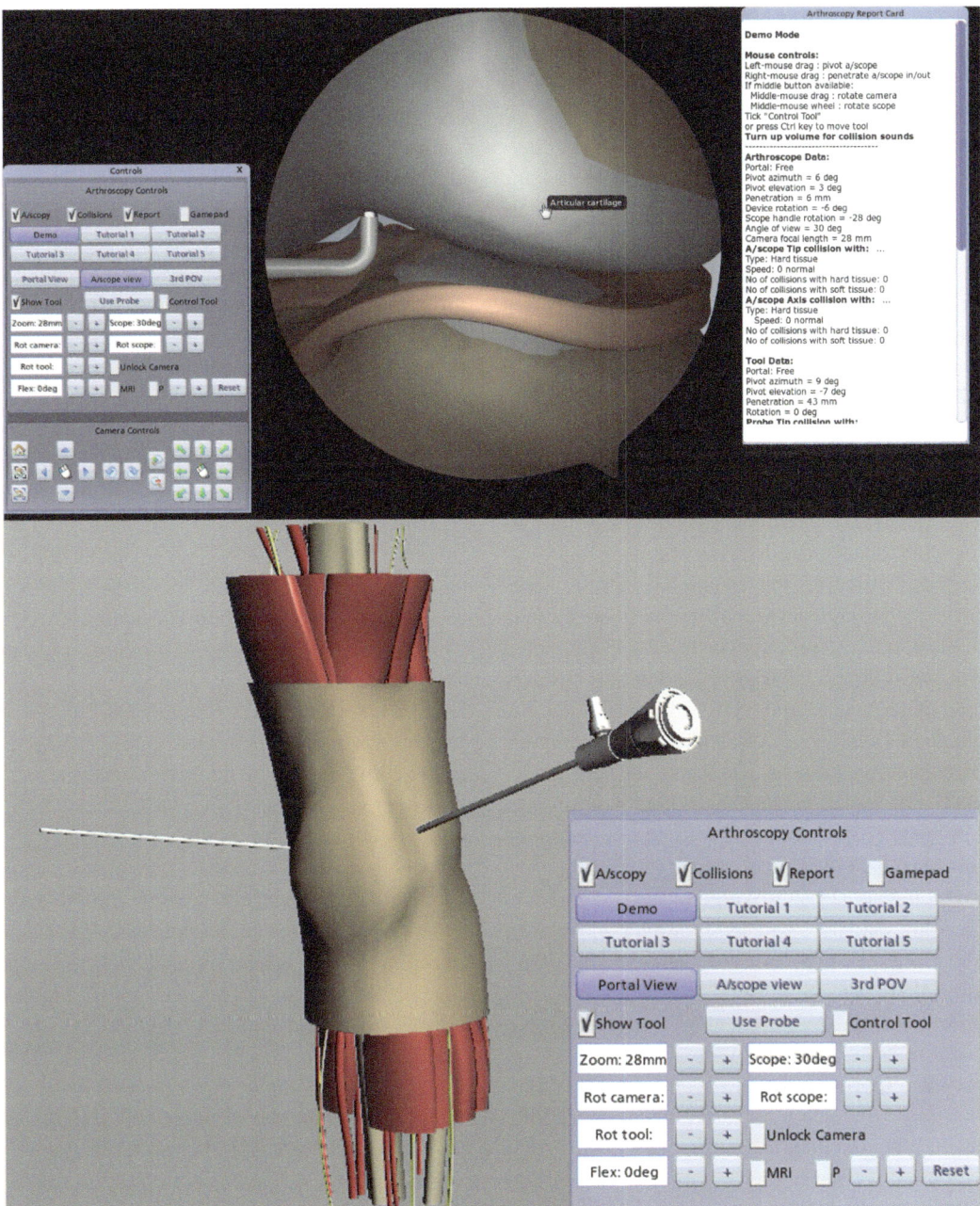

Fig. 4.1 Screenshot of VATMAS online simulator and screenshot of Epicardio simulator (© K Sherman, 2014. Reprinted with permission)

CRM is a management system using all available resources – equipment, procedures and people – in an optimal way to promote safety and enhance the efficiency of operations. Examples from the medical field are to indicate the importance and effectiveness of team training.

Grogan and coworkers (2004) implemented an 8 h CRM training course and the participants indicated that it improves attitudes towards fatigue management, team building, communication, recognising adverse events, team decision-making and performance feedback. Participants indicated that CRM training will reduce errors and improve patient safety. Neily and coworkers (2010) showed that team training reduces surgical mortality with 18 %.

France and coworkers (2008) performed direct observational analyses on 30 surgical teams and evaluated surgical team compliance with integrated safety and CRM practices after extensive CRM training. They found that the observed surgical teams were compliant with only 60 % of the CRM and perioperative safety practices emphasised in the training programme. The results highlight the challenge to adapt CRM from aviation to medicine. Although several organisations offer CRM training to health care professionals, CRM training is currently not yet part of standard education.

Operating room assistants and anaesthesiology personnel already have implemented such training; however, this is lagging behind somewhat in the surgical specialities. Disconnection in perception of teamwork in the operating room was reported previously by Sexton and coworkers (2000), who studied 1,033 operating room personnel (surgeons, anaesthesiologists, surgical residents, anaesthesia residents, surgical nurses and anaesthesia nurses). A majority of surgical residents (73 %) and surgeons (64 %) reported high levels of teamwork, but only 39 % of anaesthesiologists, 28 % of surgical nurses, 25 % of anaesthesia nurses and 10 % of anaesthesia residents reported high levels of teamwork. So in this area, there is much to gain.

4.4.2 Communication

Failure in communication has been identified as one of main contributing factors in adverse events (Kohn et al. 2000). Gawande and coworkers (2003) reported that after interviewing surgeons, 43 % of adverse events were a direct result of communication failures. Lingard and coworkers (2004) found 129 communication failures during 421 analysed relevant communication events (~30 %). They classified the communications into four different types: (1) occasion (45.7 %), in which timing of an exchange was requested or provided too late to be useful; (2) content (35.7 %),

in which information was missing or inaccurate; (3) purpose (24.0 %), in which issues were not resolved; and (4) audience (20.9 %), in which key individuals were excluded. In 36 % of these communication failures, visible effects on system processes were found, such as inefficiency, team tension, resource waste, workaround, delay, patient inconvenience and procedural error. They indicated that these weaknesses in communication in the operating room may derive from a lack of standardisation and team integration.

Principles of crew resource management techniques can be applied to the operating room to improve communication. Awad and coworkers (2005) showed that medical team training using crew resource management along with the use of a change team can improve communication in the operating room through the use of preoperative briefings. Perceptions of communication between anaesthesia and surgery were improved significantly.

4.4.3 Leadership

Leadership in surgery entails professionalism, technical competence, motivation, innovation, teamwork, communication skills, decision-making, business acumen, emotional competence, resilience and effective teaching. Leadership skills can be developed through experience, observation and education using a framework including mentoring, coaching, networking, stretch assignments, action learning and feedback (Patel et al. 2010). Leadership is not formally taught at any level in surgical training; there are no mandatory leadership courses or qualifications for trainees or specialists, and leadership performance is rarely evaluated within surgical appraisal or assessment programmes. Therefore, it is imperative that leadership programmes are implemented in medical education curriculum and postgraduate surgical training (Patel et al. 2010).

4.4.4 Situation Awareness

Situation awareness (SA) is the perception of elements in the environment within a volume of time and space, the comprehension of their meaning and the projection of their status in the near future. It involves being aware of what is happening in the vicinity, in order to understand how information, events and one's own actions will impact goals and objectives, both immediately and in the near future (Endsley 1995). Hogan and coworkers developed a novel assessment technique for practical trauma education and used the human patient simulator available in trauma education. Hogan used the Situation Awareness Global Assessment Technique (SAGAT) which has been widely used in other fields interested in performance in intense, dynamic situations and found it to be a valid, reliable measure of situation awareness (Hogan et al. 2006). They showed that information provided by SAGAT could provide specific feedback, direct individualised teaching and support curriculum change.

4.4.5 Simulation Training for Team Skills

Paige and coworkers (2009) measured the effect after all general surgical operating room team members at an academic affiliated medical centre underwent scenario-based training using a mobile mock operating room. They found that high-fidelity, simulation-based operating room team training at the point of care positively impacts 4 of the 16 items rated. They found that it improves self-efficacy for effective teamwork performance in everyday practice. Undre and coworkers found that multidisciplinary simulation-based team training is feasible (Undre et al. 2007). The differences in performance found indicate where there is a need for further training. The training was well received by surgical teams. They used human observers to assess non-technical skills. Issues that still need attention are the team performance measures for training: what to assess and how to assess. Furthermore, the development and evaluation of systematic training for technical and non-technical skills to enhance team performance are still in an early stage of development.

4.4.6 Integration of Skills and Knowledge

The independence digital media allows from the classroom to makes it easy and attractive to implement problem-based learning and lifelong learning strategies in the workplace (Obdeijn et al. 2014). Knowledge acquisition, procedural/technical skills training and team skills training have different requirements and are practised in different settings. For example, e-learning-based knowledge acquisition can be flexibly scheduled and private, whereas team skills training is bound to a specific setting and requires coordinating multiple participants. Before the resident is ready to continue training in the operating room, these different skills need to be integrated. Cognitive apprenticeship provides an approach to do just that.

4.4.7 Cognitive Apprenticeship

Cognitive apprenticeship takes into account that learned skills are performed in a specific professional context, and since many performance rules may be implicit in such an environment, training should be located in a similar context (Brown et al. 1989). Also, expert performance is often automated to a degree that an expert will find it

> *Modelling*: This involves the expert performing the skill so that the trainee can observe and build a conceptual model of the processes required to accomplish it.
> *Coaching*: Here, the expert observes the trainee perform the skill and offers hints, feedback, reminders and perhaps further modelling – aimed at bringing the trainee's performance closer to that of the expert.
> *Scaffolding*: Learning is supported according to current skill level, and activities are organised to assist the trainee to progress to the next level. Support is gradually removed (fading) until the trainee is able to accomplish the skill alone.

Articulation: This involves any method of assisting the trainee to articulate their knowledge, reasoning, or problem-solving processes, e.g. questioning, explaining what they are doing and why they do it that way.

Reflection: Enabling the trainee to be critical of their own performance and problem-solving processes and to compare these with those of an expert, another trainee and, ultimately, an internal cognitive model of expertise.

Exploration: This involves pushing students into a mode of problem-solving on their own – critical if trainees are to adapt to new problems in the real world.

hard to formulate important performance principles. In contrast to traditional master-apprentice training, cognitive apprenticeship aims to structure learning in such a way that implicit rules and performance aspects are made explicit. To create a learning environment based on cognitive apprenticeship principles, the following six techniques need to be applied (Collins et al. as quoted in Woolley and Jarvis (2007)):

By explicitly aiming to simulate the whole professional context (including practical skills, knowledge and team skills), and by its structured, analytical approach to build towards competency by integrating these diverse subskills, cognitive apprenticeship is well suited to prepare the resident for the transition to continued training in the operating room.

Bibliography

Adams JA (1971) A closed-loop theory of motor learning. J Mot Behav 3(2):111–149, available from: PM:15155169

Allum R (2002) Complications of arthroscopy of the knee. J Bone Joint Surg Br 84(7):937–945, available from: PM:12358382

Alvand A, Auplish S, Gill H, Rees J (2011) Innate arthroscopic skills in medical students and variation in learning curves. J Bone Joint Surg Am 93(19):e115–e119, available from: PM:22005876

American Board of Internal Medicine (1991) Guide to evaluation of residents in internal medicine, 1991–1992. American Board of Internal Medicine, Philadelphia

Amrein A, Berliner D (2002) High-stakes testing & student learning. Educ Policy Anal Arch 10:18

Anderson LW, Kratwohl DR, Airasian PW, Cruikshank KA, Mayer RE, Pintrich PR, Raths J, Wittrock MC (2001) A taxonomy for learning, teaching, and assessing: a revision of Bloom's taxonomy of educational objectives. Pearson, Allyn & Bacon, New York

Atesok K, Mabrey JD, Jazrawi LM, Egol KA (2012) Surgical simulation in orthopaedic skills training. J Am Acad Orthop Surg 20(7):410–422, available from: PM:22751160

Awad SS, Fagan SP, Bellows C, Albo D, Green-Rashad B, De la Garza M, Berger DH (2005) Bridging the communication gap in the operating room with medical team training. Am J Surg 190(5):770–774, available from: PM:16226956

Bell RH Jr (2004) Alternative training models for surgical residency. Surg Clin North Am 84(6):1699–1711, xii available from: PM:15501282

Bholat OS, Haluck RS, Murray WB, Gorman PJ, Krummel TM (1999) Tactile feedback is present during minimally invasive surgery. J Am Coll Surg 189(4):349–355, available from: PM:10509459

Biggs J (2003) Constructing learning by aligning teaching: constructive alignment. In: Biggs J (ed) Teaching for quality learning at university, 2nd edn. Open University Press, Berkshire, pp 11–33

Bloom BS, Engelhart MD, Furst EJ, Hill WH, Kratwohl DR (1956) Taxonomy of educational objectives, the classification of educational goals – Handbook I: cognitive domain. McKay, New York

Boyle E, Al-Akash M, Gallagher AG, Traynor O, Hill AD, Neary PC (2011) Optimising surgical training: use of feedback to reduce errors during a simulated surgical procedure. Postgrad Med J 87(1030):524–528, available from: PM:21642446

Braun DA, Aertsen A, Wolpert DM, Mehring C (2009) Motor task variation induces structural learning. Curr Biol 19(4):352–357, available from: PM:19217296

Braun DA, Mehring C, Wolpert DM (2010) Structure learning in action. Behav Brain Res 206(2):157–165, available from: PM:19720086

Brown J, Collins A, Duguid P (1989) Situated cognition and the culture of learning. Educ Res 18(1):32–42

Castricini R, De BM, Orlando N, Rocchi M, Zini R, Pirani P (2013) Arthroscopic Latarjet procedure: analysis of the learning curve. Musculoskelet Surg 97(Suppl 1):93–98, available from: PM:23588833

Chami G, Ward JW, Phillips R, Sherman KP (2008) Haptic feedback can provide an objective assessment of arthroscopic skills. Clin Orthop Relat Res 466(4):963–968, available from: PM:18213507

Clark R, Mayer R (2011) E-learning and the science of instruction: proven guidelines for consumers and designers of multimedia learning, 3rd edn. John Wiley & Sons, Pfeiffer

Commission of the European Communities. Adult learning: it is never too late to learn. http://europa.eu/legislation_summaries/education_training_youth/lifelong_learning/c11097_en.htm. Updated 2007. Accessed 30 May 2014

Committee on Ethics and Standards and the Board of Directors of the Arthroscopy Association of North America (2008) Suggested guidelines for the practice of arthroscopic surgery. Arthroscopy 24(6):A30, available from: PM:18536081

Cullen KA, Hall MJ, Golosinskiy A (2009) Ambulatory surgery in the United States, 2006. Natl Health Stat Report (11):1–25 available from: PM:19294964

Dankelman J, Chmarra MK, Verdaasdonk EG, Stassen LP, Grimbergen CA (2005) Fundamental aspects of learning minimally invasive surgical skills. Minim Invasive Ther Allied Technol 14(4):247–256, available from: PM:16754171

Dave RH (1970) Psychomotor levels. In: Armstrong RJ (ed) Developing and writing behavioral objectives. Educational Innovators Press, Tucson

Davidson PR, Wolpert DM (2003) Motor learning and prediction in a variable environment. Curr Opin Neurobiol 13(2):232–237, available from: PM:12744979

Dawson SL, Kaufman JA (1998) The imperative for medical simulation. Proc IEEE 86(3):479–483, available from: ISI:000072454200003

Endsley MR (1995) Toward a theory of situation awareness in dynamic-systems. Hum Factors 37(1):32–64, available from: ISI:A1995RL73500004

Eversbusch A, Grantcharov TP (2004) Learning curves and impact of psychomotor training on performance in simulated colonoscopy: a randomized trial using a virtual reality endoscopy trainer. Surg Endosc 18(10):1514–1518, available from: PM:15791380

Fitts PM, Posner MI (1967) Human performance. Brooks/Cole, Belmont

Flanagan JR, Vetter P, Johansson RS, Wolpert DM (2003) Prediction precedes control in motor learning. Curr Biol 13(2):146–150, available from: PM:12546789

France DJ, Leming-Lee S, Jackson T, Feistritzer NR, Higgins MS (2008) An observational analysis of surgical team compliance with perioperative safety practices after crew resource management training. Am J Surg 195(4):546–553, available from: PM:18304501

Frank RM, Erickson B, Frank JM, Bush-Joseph CA, Bach BR Jr, Cole BJ, Romeo AA, Provencher MT, Verma NN (2014) Utility of modern arthroscopic simulator training models. Arthroscopy 30(1):121–133, available from: PM:24290789

Gagne R (1965) The conditions of learning. Holt, Rinehart and Winston. Inc, New York

Gallagher AG, Ritter EM, Lederman AB, McClusky DA III, Smith CD (2005) Video-assisted surgery represents more than a loss of three-dimensional vision. Am J Surg 189(1):76–80, available from: PM:15701497

Gallagher AG, Leonard G, Traynor OJ (2009) Role and feasibility of psychomotor and dexterity testing in selection for surgical training. ANZ J Surg 79(3):108–113, available from: PM:19317772

Gallagher AG, Jordan-Black JA, O'Sullivan GC (2012) Prospective, randomized assessment of the acquisition, maintenance, and loss of laparoscopic skills. Ann Surg 256(2):387–393, available from: PM:22580935

Gardner H (2011) Frames of mind: the theory of multiple intelligences, 3rd edn. Basic Books, New York

Garrett WE Jr, Swiontkowski MF, Weinstein JN, Callaghan J, Rosier RN, Berry DJ, Harrast J, Derosa GP (2006) American Board of Orthopaedic Surgery Practice of the Orthopaedic Surgeon: Part-II, certification examination case mix. J Bone Joint Surg Am 88(3):660–667, available from: PM:16510834

Gawande AA, Zinner MJ, Studdert DM, Brennan TA (2003) Analysis of errors reported by surgeons at three teaching hospitals. Surgery 133(6):614–621, available from: PM:12796727

Georgoulis A, Randelli P (2011) Education in arthroscopy, sports medicine and knee surgery. Knee Surg Sports Traumatol Arthrosc 19(8):1231–1232, available from: PM:21630049

Gomoll AH, Pappas G, Forsythe B, Warner JJ (2008) Individual skill progression on a virtual reality simulator for shoulder arthroscopy: a 3-year follow-up study. Am J Sports Med 36(6):1139–1142, available from: PM:18326032

Grechenig W, Fellinger M, Fankhauser F, Weiglein AH (1999) The Graz learning and training model for arthroscopic surgery. Surg Radiol Anat 21(5):347–350, available from: PM:10635100

Grogan EL, Stiles RA, France DJ, Speroff T, Morris JA Jr, Nixon B, Gaffney FA, Seddon R, Pinson CW (2004) The impact of aviation-based teamwork training on the attitudes of health-care professionals. J Am Coll Surg 199(6):843–848, available from: PM:15555963

Hall MP, Kaplan KM, Gorczynski CT, Zuckerman JD, Rosen JE (2010) Assessment of arthroscopic training in U.S. orthopedic surgery residency program-- resident self-assessment. Bull NYU Hosp Jt Dis 68(1):5–10, available from: PM:20345354

Hanna GB, Shimi SM, Cuschieri A (1998) Randomised study of influence of two-dimensional versus three-dimensional imaging on performance of laparoscopic cholecystectomy. Lancet 351(9098):248–251, available from: PM:9457094

Harewood GC, Murray F, Winder S, Patchett S (2008) Evaluation of formal feedback on endoscopic competence among trainees: the EFFECT trial. Ir J Med Sci 177(3):253–256, available from: PM:18584274

Hawes R, Lehman GA, Hast J, O'Connor KW, Crabb DW, Lui A, Christiansen PA (1986) Training resident physicians in fiberoptic sigmoidoscopy. How many supervised examinations are required to achieve competence? Am J Med 80(3):465–470, available from: PM:3953621

Hmelo-Silver CE (2004) Problem-based learning: what and how do students learn? Educ Psychol Rev 16(3):235–266, available from: ISI:000222473700003

Hogan MP, Pace DE, Hapgood J, Boone DC (2006) Use of human patient simulation and the situation awareness global assessment technique in practical trauma skills assessment. J Trauma 61(5):1047–1052, available from: PM:17099507

Hoppe DJ, de SD, Simunovic N, Bhandari M, Safran MR, Larson CM, Ayeni OR (2014) The learning curve for hip arthroscopy: a systematic review. Arthroscopy 30:389–397, available from: PM:24461140

Horeman T, Rodrigues SP, van den Dobbelsteen JJ, Jansen FW, Dankelman J (2012) Visual force feedback in laparoscopic training. Surg Endosc 26(1):242–248, available from: PM:21858573

Horton W (2011) E-learning by design, 2nd edn. Wiley & Sons, Pfeiffer

Hui Y, Safir O, Dubrowski A, Carnahan H (2013) What skills should simulation training in arthroscopy teach residents? A focus on resident input. Int J Comput Assist Radiol Surg 8:945–953, available from: PM:23535939

Hurmusiadis V, Rhode K, Schaeffter T, Sherman K (2011) Virtual arthroscopy trainer for minimally invasive surgery. Stud Health Technol Inform 163:236–238, available from: PM:21335795

Jonassen D (1999) Designing constructivist learning environments. Instr Des Theor Models New Paradigm Instr Theory 2:215–239

Karahan M, Unalan PC, Bozkurt S, Odabas I, Akgun U, Cifcili S, Lobenhoffer P, Aydin AT (2009) Correlation of basic motor skills with arthroscopic experience. Acta Orthop Traumatol Turc 43(1):49–53, available from: PM:19293616

Kaufman HH, Wiegand RL, Tunick RH (1987) Teaching surgeons to operat--rinciples of psychomotor skills training. Acta Neurochir (Wien) 87(1–2):1–7, available from: PM:3314366

Kawato M (1999) Internal models for motor control and trajectory planning. Curr Opin Neurobiol 9(6):718–727, available from: PM:10607637

Kim RH, Gilbert T, Ristig K, Chu QD (2013) Surgical resident learning styles: faculty and resident accuracy at identification of preferences and impact on ABSITE scores. J Surg Res 184(1):31–36, available from: PM:23706561

Kocher RJ, Nicandri GT (2013) Using the arthroscopic surgery skill evaluation tool as a pass-fail examination. J Bone Joint Surg Am 95(23):e1871–e1876, available from: PM:24306710

Kohn L, Corrigan J, Donaldson M (2000) To err is human: building a safer health system. National Academy Press, Washington DC

Kording KP, Wolpert DM (2004) Bayesian integration in sensorimotor learning. Nature 427(6971):244–247, available from: PM:14724638

Leonard M, Kennedy J, Kiely P, Murphy P (2007) Knee arthroscopy: how much training is necessary? A cross-sectional study. Eur J Orthop Surg Traumatol 17:359–362

Lingard L, Espin S, Whyte S, Regehr G, Baker GR, Reznick R, Bohnen J, Orser B, Doran D, Grober E (2004) Communication failures in the operating room: an observational classification of recurrent types and effects. Qual Saf Health Care 13(5):330–334, available from: PM:15465935

Megali G, Tonet O, Dario P, Vascellari A, Marcacci M (2005) Computer-assisted training system for knee arthroscopy. Int J Med Robot 1(3):57–66, available from: PM:17518391

Merriam S, Caffarella R, Baumgartner L (2012) Learning in adulthood: a comprehensive guide. John Wiley & Sons, New York

Merrienboer J, Clark S, Croock M (2002) Blueprints for complex learning: the 4C/ID-model. Educ Tech Res Develop 50:39–64

Miller WE (1985) Learning arthroscopy. South Med J 78(8):935–937, available from: PM:4023785

Modi CS, Morris G, Mukherjee R (2010) Computer-simulation training for knee and shoulder arthroscopic surgery. Arthroscopy 26(6):832–840, available from: PM:20511043

Morris AH, Jennings JE, Stone RG, Katz JA, Garroway RY, Hendler RC (1993) Guidelines for privileges in arthroscopic surgery. Arthroscopy 9(1):125–127, available from: PM:8442822

Neequaye SK, Aggarwal R, Brightwell R, Van Herzeele I, Darzi A, Cheshire NJ (2007) Identification of skills common to renal and iliac endovascular procedures performed on a virtual reality simulator. Eur J Vasc Endovasc Surg 33(5):525–532, available from: PM:17291792

Neily J, Mills PD, Young-Xu Y, Carney BT, West P, Berger DH, Mazzia LM, Paull DE, Bagian JP (2010) Association between implementation of a medical team training program and surgical mortality. JAMA 304(15):1693–1700, available from: PM:20959579

Neiman Z (1989) Teaching specific motor skills for conducting to young music students. Percept Mot Skills 68(3 Pt 1):847–858, available from: PM:2748301

O'Connor A, Schwaitzberg SD, Cao CG (2008) How much feedback is necessary for learning to suture? Surg Endosc 22(7):1614–1619, available from: PM:17973165

O'Neill PJ, Cosgarea AJ, Freedman JA, Queale WS, McFarland EG (2002) Arthroscopic proficiency: a survey of orthopaedic sports medicine fellowship directors and orthopaedic surgery department chairs. Arthroscopy 18(7):795–800, available from: PM:12209439

Obdeijn MC, Bavinck N, Mathoulin C, van der Horst CM, Schijven MP, Tuijthof GJ (2013) Education in wrist arthroscopy: past, present and future. Knee Surg Sports Traumatol Arthrosc. available from: PM:23835770

Obdeijn MC, Alewijnse JV, Mathoulin C, Liverneaux P, Tuijthof GJ, Schijven MP (2014) Development and validation of a computer-based learning module for wrist arthroscopy. Chir Main 33:100–105, available from: PM:24560535

Omrod J, Davis K (2004) Human learning. Merrill, London

Oxford English Dictionary. Oxford University Press. http://www.oed.com/. Accessed 15 Jan 2014

Paige JT, Kozmenko V, Yang T, Paragi GR, Hilton CW, Cohn I Jr, Chauvin SW (2009) High-fidelity, simulation-based, interdisciplinary operating room team training at the point of care. Surgery 145(2):138–146, available from: PM:19167968

Paris S, Winograd P (1990) How metacognition can promote academic learning and instruction. Dimens Think Cogn Instr 1:15–51

Patel VM, Warren O, Humphris P, Ahmed K, Ashrafian H, Rao C, Athanasiou T, Darzi A (2010) What does leadership in surgery entail? ANZ J Surg 80(12):876–883, available from: PM:21114726

Pedowitz RA, Esch J, Snyder S (2002) Evaluation of a virtual reality simulator for arthroscopy skills development. Arthroscopy 18(6):E29, available from: PM:12098111

Pories W (1999) Some reflections on Halsted and residency training. Curr Surg 56(1–2):1

Rovai AP, Wighting MJ, Baker JD, Grooms LD (2009) Development of an instrument to measure perceived cognitive, affective, and psychomotor learning in traditional and virtual classroom higher education settings. Internet Higher Educ 12(1):7–13, available from: ISI:000264833900002

Safir O, Dubrowski A, Mirsky L, Lin C, Backstein D, Carnahan A (2008) What skills should simulation training in arthroscopy teach residents? Int J Comput Assist Radiol Surg 3(5):433–437

Schaafsma BE, Hiemstra E, Dankelman J, Jansen FW (2009) Feedback in laparoscopic skills acquisition: an observational study during a basic skills training course. Gynecol Surg 6(4):339–343, available from: PM:20234844

Sealy W (1999) Halsted is dead: time for change in graduate surgical education. Curr Surg 56(1–2):34–38

Seidler RD (2007) Older adults can learn to learn new motor skills. Behav Brain Res 183(1):118–122, available from: PM:17602760

Sexton JB, Thomas EJ, Helmreich RL (2000) Error, stress, and teamwork in medicine and aviation: cross sectional surveys. BMJ 320(7237):745–749, available from: PM:10720356

Shadmehr R, Smith MA, Krakauer JW (2010) Error correction, sensory prediction, and adaptation in motor control. Annu Rev Neurosci 33:89–108, available from: PM:20367317

Shearer CB (1998) MIDAS: Multiple Intelligences Developmental Assessment Scales, Adult Version. Corwin, USA

Sherman KP, Ward JW, Wills DP, Sherman VJ, Mohsen AM (2001) Surgical trainee assessment using a VE knee arthroscopy training system (VE-KATS): experimental results. Stud Health Technol Inform 81:465–470, available from: PM:11317792

Simpson EJ (1972) The classification of educational objectives in the psychomotor domain. Gryphon House, Washington, DC

Slade Shantz JA, Leiter JR, Gottschalk T, MacDonald PB (2014) The internal validity of arthroscopic simulators and their effectiveness in arthroscopic education. Knee Surg Sports Traumatol Arthrosc 22(1):33–40, available from: PM:23052120

Smeets JB, van den Dobbelsteen JJ, de Grave DD, van Beers RJ, Brenner E (2006) Sensory integration does not lead to sensory calibration. Proc Natl Acad Sci U S A 103(49):18781–18786, available from: PM:17130453

Straub RO, Terrace HS (1981) Generalization of serial-learning in the pigeon. Anim Learn Behav 9(4):454–468, available from: ISI:A1981MZ83400003

Strom P, Kjellin A, Hedman L, Wredmark T, Fellander-Tsai L (2004) Training in tasks with different visual-spatial components does not improve virtual arthroscopy performance. Surg Endosc 18(1):115–120, available from: PM:14625735

Suggested guidelines for the practice of arthroscopic surgery (2008). Arthroscopy, 24, (6) A30 available from: PM:18536081

Suksudaj N, Townsend GC, Kaidonis J, Lekkas D, Winning TA (2012) Acquiring psychomotor skills in operative dentistry: do innate ability and motivation matter? Eur J Dent Educ 16(1):e187–e194, available from: PM:22251344

Sulzenbruck S, Heuer H (2012) Enhanced mechanical transparency during practice impedes open-loop control of a complex tool. Exp Brain Res 218(2):283–294, available from: PM:22278111

Thomas W (2008) The making of a surgeon. Surgery (Oxford) 26(10):400–402

Tokuhama-Espinosa T (2010) Mind, brain, and education science: a comprehensive guide to the new brain-based teaching, 1st edn. W.W. Norton & Company Inc, New York

Triano JJ, Scaringe J, Bougie J, Rogers C (2006) Effects of visual feedback on manipulation performance and patient ratings. J Manipulative Physiol Ther 29(5):378–385, available from: PM:16762666

Tuijthof GJ, Visser P, Sierevelt IN, van Dijk CN, Kerkhoffs GM (2011) Does perception of usefulness of arthroscopic simulators differ with levels of experience? Clin Orthop Relat Res 469:1701–1708, available from: PM:21290203

Unalan PC, Akan K, Orhun H, Akgun U, Poyanli O, Baykan A, Yavuz Y, Beyzadeoglu T, Nuran R, Kocaoglu B, Topsakal N, Akman M, Karahan M (2010) A basic arthroscopy course based on motor skill training. Knee Surg Sports Traumatol Arthrosc 18(10):1395–1399, available from: PM:20012013

Undre S, Koutantji M, Sevdalis N, Gautama S, Selvapatt N, Williams S, Sains P, McCulloch P, Darzi A, Vincent C (2007) Multidisciplinary crisis simulations: the way forward for training surgical teams. World J Surg 31(9):1843–1853, available from: PM:17610109

van Beers RJ (2009) Motor learning is optimally tuned to the properties of motor noise. Neuron 63(3):406–417, available from: PM:19679079

Verdaasdonk EG, Stassen LP, Schijven MP, Dankelman J (2007) Construct validity and assessment of the learning curve for the SIMENDO endoscopic simulator. Surg Endosc 21(8):1406–1412, available from: PM:17653815

Vitale MA, Kleweno CP, Jacir AM, Levine WN, Bigliani LU, Ahmad CS (2007) Training resources in arthroscopic rotator cuff repair. J Bone Joint Surg Am 89(6):1393–1398, available from: PM:17545443

Wanzel KR, Ward M, Reznick RK (2002) Teaching the surgical craft: from selection to certification. Curr Probl Surg 39(6):573–659, available from: PM:12037512

Wentink M, Breedveld P, Stassen LP, Oei IH, Wieringa PA (2002) A clearly visible endoscopic instrument shaft on the monitor facilitates hand-eye coordination. Surg Endosc 16(11):1533–1537, available from: PM:12072991

Windsor JA, Diener S, Zoha F (2008) Learning style and laparoscopic experience in psychomotor skill performance using a virtual reality surgical simulator. Am J Surg 195(6):837–842, available from: PM:18417084

Wirth K, Malone B, Barrera K, Widmann WD, Turner C, Sanni A (2014) Is there a place for medical students as teachers in the education of junior residents? Am J Surg 207(2):271–274, available from: PM:24468027

Wolpert DM, Ghahramani Z (2000) Computational principles of movement neuroscience. Nat Neurosci 3(Suppl):1212–1217, available from: PM:11127840

Wolpert DM, Miall RC (1996) Forward models for physiological motor control. Neural Netw 9(8):1265–1279, available from: PM:12662535

Woolley NN, Jarvis Y (2007) Situated cognition and cognitive apprenticeship: a model for teaching and learning clinical skills in a technologically rich and authentic learning environment. Nurse Educ Today 27(1):73–79, available from: PM:16624452

Part II

Simulated Environments

Traditional Wet Labs and Industry Involvement

5

Amelie Stoehr, Mustafa Karahan, and Hermann O. Mayr

Take-Home Messages

- Many options exist to train arthroscopic techniques before training on patients is started. Cadaver training is popular as the material is most similar to arthroscopy in patients. Therefore, it should be an obligatory part in the education of arthroscopic surgeons.
- For cost efficiency, cadaver training can be performed in cooperation with industry, but care has to be taken that they do not influence the training content.
- Arthroscopy training on animal models can be helpful in the beginning of curriculum.

A. Stoehr (✉)
Department of Knee Surgery and Sports
Traumatology, Gem-Clinic, Munich, Germany
e-mail: ameliestoehr@hotmail.de

M. Karahan
Department of Orthopedics and Traumatology,
Acibadem University School of Medicine,
Istanbul, Turkey
e-mail: drmustafakarahan@gmail.com

H.O. Mayr, MD
Department of Orthopedic and Trauma Surgery,
Albert Ludwig University of Freiburg,
Freiburg, Germany
e-mail: hermann.mayr.ocm@gmx.de

5.1 Introduction

An increasing number of all operative procedures in orthopedic surgery are performed arthroscopically (Pedowitz et al. 2002). Simultaneously, there are a steadily rising number of residents. The task is to maintain high-quality standards and to guarantee an adequate training in arthroscopic surgery (Morris et al. 1993). Fortunately, arthroscopic skills can be partially trained in laboratory settings using artificial models and cadaver joints with experienced surgeons and anatomists acting as supervisors (Wolf and Britton 2013) and with instructors that guarantee sufficient practical experience during the training period (Grechenig et al. 1999). Orthopedic trainees indicate that they highly benefit from arthroscopic skills teaching in labs or special courses (Wolf and Britton 2013) using cadaver material. To monitor training progress, objective evaluation tools have been developed for in-training evaluations and to measure the impact of skills curricula (see elaboration on evaluation tools in Chap. 13) (Butler et al. 2013; Slade Shantz et al. 2013). This chapter will focus on the use of cadavers – both animal and human – for training.

5.2 Animal Cadavers

In literature, bovine and porcine animal models of the knee and shoulder have been developed to train arthroscopy (Mattos e Dinato et al. 2010;

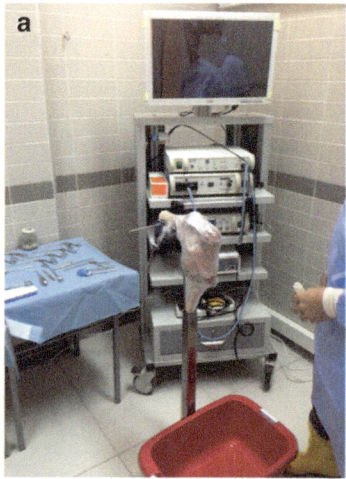 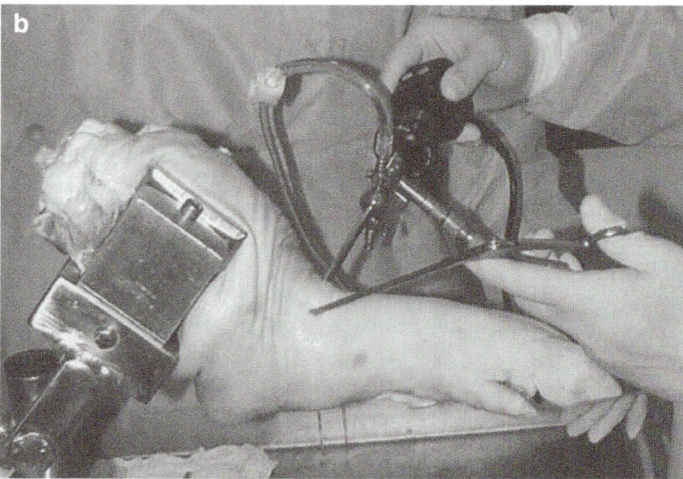

Fig. 5.1 (**a**) Wet lab setup for training with a bovine knee (Unalan et al. 2010). (**b**) Wet lab setup for training with a porcine ankle (Mattos e Dinato 2010, copyright © 2010 by (Copyright Holder). Reprinted by Permission of SAGE Publications)

Patel and Guhl 1983; Splawski 2011; Unalan et al. 2010; Voto et al. 1988). Both animal species present a similar gross and arthroscopic anatomy as the human knee joint. In the early 1980s, Patel and Guhl proposed to use a bovine knee (Patel and Guhl 1983). Unalan and coworkers (Unalan et al. 2010) have further developed this means of simulated training and incorporated this in their basic arthroscopy course, which consists of six steps. In this wet lab step, basic arthroscopic procedures such as diagnosis, synovectomy, loose body extraction, meniscectomy, and microfracture can be completed by the guidance of an instructor (Fig. 5.1). To mimic an arthroscopic procedure with the use of bovine knees they need to be prepared. The bovine knees have extensions of 20–25 cm to the proximal and distal parts; are stripped of all soft tissue, especially the Hoffa pad; and are covered with stretch film to allow fluid irrigation during training.

Similar as the bovine specimens, porcine knees, ankles, and shoulders also need to be prepared before training can take place (Fig. 5.1). This involves leaving part of the proximal and distal long bones attached for fixation, proper positioning in holders, and removal of muscles externally surrounding the joint (Mattos e Dinato et al. 2010; Splawski 2011; Voto et al. 1988). Training can take place using normal arthroscopic

equipment and implants can be reused after training. Voto and coworkers also mention the use of canine knees and horse ankles that can be used for arthroscopy training, but no literature was found describing this (Voto et al. 1988).

5.3 Human Cadavers

As indicated in Chap. 2, human cadaver joints are preferred both by teaching staff and residents as means to perform skills lab training (Hui et al. 2013; Safir et al. 2008; Vitale et al. 2007; Wolf and Britton 2013). Human cadavers are the most realistic mode of simulation for arthroscopic training (Madan and Pai 2014). Both fresh frozen and embalmed cadavers have been used in arthroscopic training. For arthroscopy training, fresh frozen cadaver joints are preferably used, but new soft-embalming techniques maintain tissue properties and preserve joint movements and can also be applied (Madan and Pai 2014). In principle, all major joints such as the knee, shoulder, hip, elbow, wrist, and ankle can be treated arthroscopically and therefore can be used for training. Most commonly offered are knee and shoulder courses. ESSKA supports several such courses and its website indicates 68 accredited training centers in Europe and one in the USA (www.esska.org).

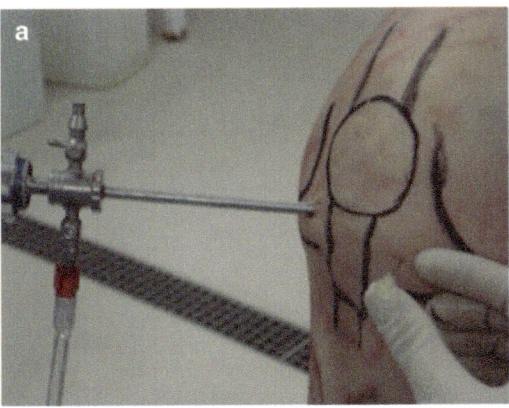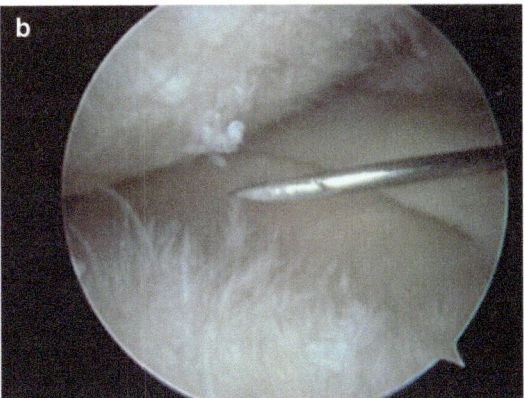

Fig. 5.2 (**a, b**) Visualizing the ventromedial arthroscopic approach to the knee using a needle (© A Stoehr, 2014. Reprinted with permission)

Novice courses teach basic knowledge and handling of arthroscopic instruments and arthroscopic exploration of the joint anatomy. Advanced courses offer training of more complex arthroscopic procedures, such as ACL reconstructions, posterior ankle arthroscopy, and shoulder stabilization techniques.

A typical setup of a novice cadaver course is as follows. The residents learn to handle the arthroscopic instruments (probe, punches, shaver, graspers) and different types of arthroscopes and to perform portal creation, three-dimensional orientation and triangulation, and manual bilateral handling of different surgical procedures. The progression in the learning curve of arthroscopic skills is slow at start, as the trainees need to adapt to the magnification factor, the two-dimensional view on the monitor, and the 30° angled field of view of the optical system. But in general, arthroscopy training reduces the number of postoperative effusion and chondral lesions due to brusque manipulation with instruments, and prolonged operating times can be minimized (Grechenig et al. 1999; Henn III et al. 2013). Failures in surgical techniques and malplacement of surgical approaches as a result of practice on cadaver joints help to protect future patients from the same mistakes. This leads to confidence and experience before continuing training in the operating room. As cadaver courses are so much preferred by teachers and trainees, it might be suggested to start participating in cadaver

courses at the end of the master in medicine program and be intensified at the beginning of residency training.

Nowadays, arthroscopy is the gold standard in treating intra-articular lesions of the human knee joint. That is why most novice courses start training of arthroscopic skills in human cadaver knees. At the beginning, external knee joint anatomy should be visualized by marking relevant structures and application of standard portal approaches (Fig. 5.2). After portal creation, a diagnostic survey is helpful to get orientation inside the intra-articular joint. Simple procedures such as partial meniscus resection (Fig. 5.3) and removal of loose bodies should be trained first, as cadaver joints from elderly can offer very tight joints which makes these basic techniques already challenging.

Advanced courses offer possibilities to practice more difficult techniques, such as meniscal repair (Fig. 5.4) and the drilling of the tunnels for the anterior and posterior cruciate ligament reconstruction with anatomically correct placement (Fig. 5.5).

Physiological ligament insertions should be assessed. Different fixation techniques can be trained to ensure experience and confidence in clinical practice.

Training of more difficult posteromedial (Fig. 5.6) and posterolateral approaches to the knee joint can safely be performed by taking into account technical options and risks of lesions of neurovascular structures (Fig. 5.7b). This is facilitated by post-training dissection of the cadaver

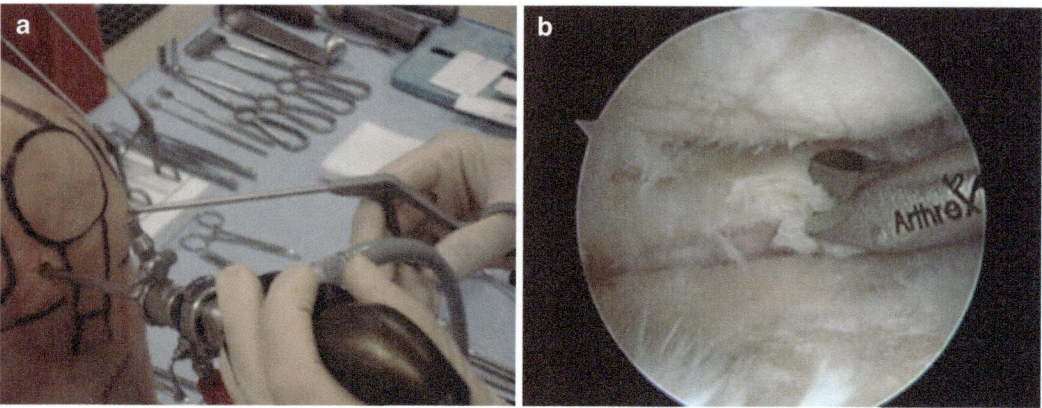

Fig. 5.3 (**a, b**) Partial meniscus resection and training of triangulation (© A Stoehr, 2014. Reprinted with permission)

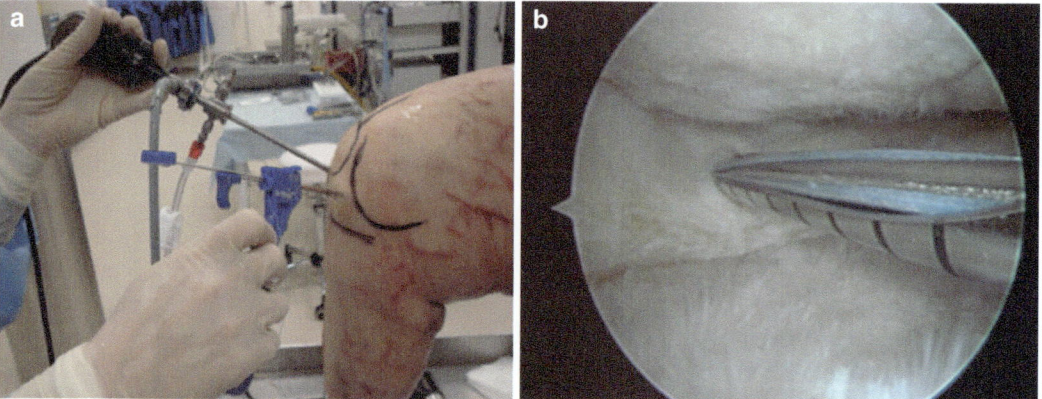

Fig. 5.4 (**a, b**) Training of meniscus suture of the posterior horn of the medial meniscus (© A Stoehr, 2014. Reprinted with permission)

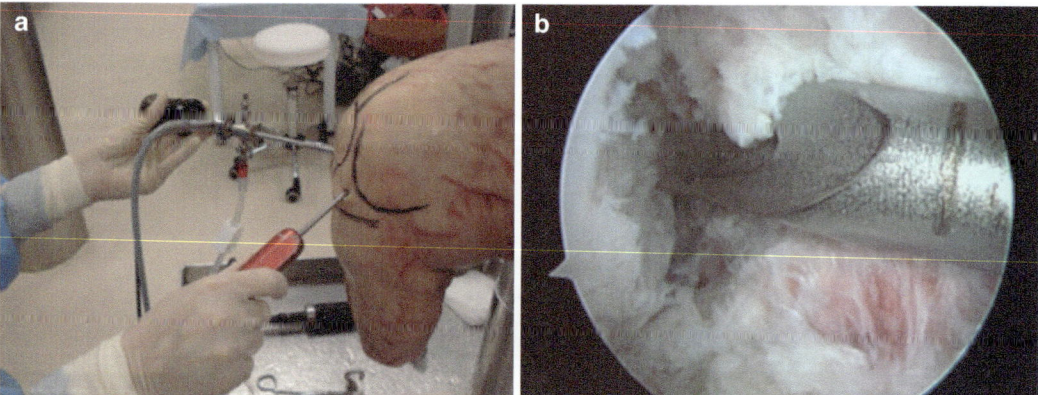

Fig. 5.5 (**a, b**) Visualizing the femoral insertion area of the anterior cruciate ligament during reconstruction (© A Stoehr, 2014. Reprinted with permission)

which involves evaluation of anatomy of neurovascular structures and their proximity to the surgical field. Also, advantages and disadvantages of various surgical access options can be studied.

In addition to practicing correct drilling of ACL and PCL tunnels, graft harvesting for ligament reconstructions can be trained (hamstrings (Fig. 5.7a), patellar tendon, and quadriceps tendon), as well as cartilage procedures, osteochondral reconstructions, and alignment procedures of the patella.

In cadaver shoulder joints, particularly the various approaches (dorsal, ventral, lateral, and cranial) to the joint and the diagnostic survey

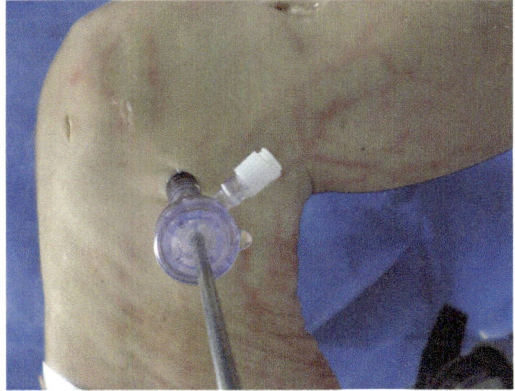

Fig. 5.6 Practice of rare posteromedial arthroscopic approach to cadaver knee. (© H Mayr, 2014. Reprinted with permission)

can be practiced. This facilitates knowledge and three-dimensional orientation of arthroscopic anatomy as all portals are created in one joint. Experience has shown that the approach to the shoulder joint is the first key point in executing in vivo shoulder arthroscopy.

Subsequently, therapeutic techniques as acromioplasty and lateral clavicular joint resection are trained (Fig. 5.8a) and again verified by post-training dissection of the cadaver as well as visualizing the neurovascular structures around the shoulder. Also, rotator cuff and Bankart repairs can be trained (Vitale et al. 2007). In comparison to the regular patient, the rotator cuff tissue is more vulnerable in cadaver joints.

There are also an increasing number of cadaver courses including hip, elbow, ankle, and wrist arthroscopy training supported by ESSKA. These are considered advanced courses and are recommended to attend after participation of the novice, advanced knee and shoulder courses.

Hip arthroscopy is a relatively new procedure. It is primarily used for the treatment of lesions (pincer/cam) in the early phases of hip joint osteoarthritis. In addition, soft tissue disorders such as lesions of the labrum and central hip band or synovial proliferations can be treated. In the hip, usually a 70° optical system is used which changes triangulation (Fig. 5.8b). Surgical

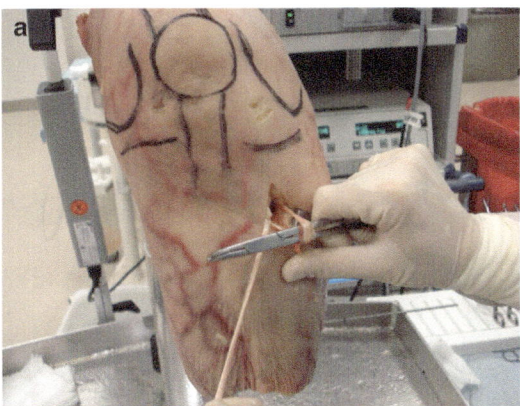
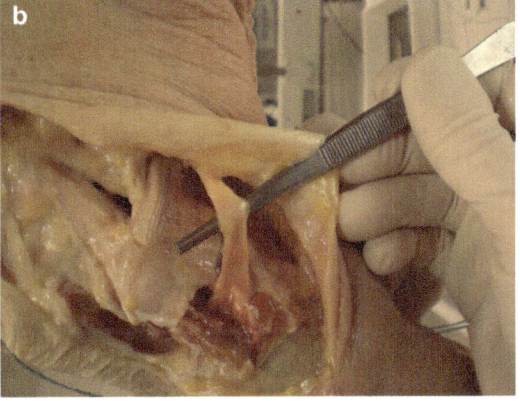

Fig. 5.7 (**a**) Harvesting of hamstring tendons (© A Stoehr, 2014. Reprinted with permission). (**b**) Open dissection of the lateral side of the knee and presentation of nervus peroneus (© H Mayr, 2014. Reprinted with permission)

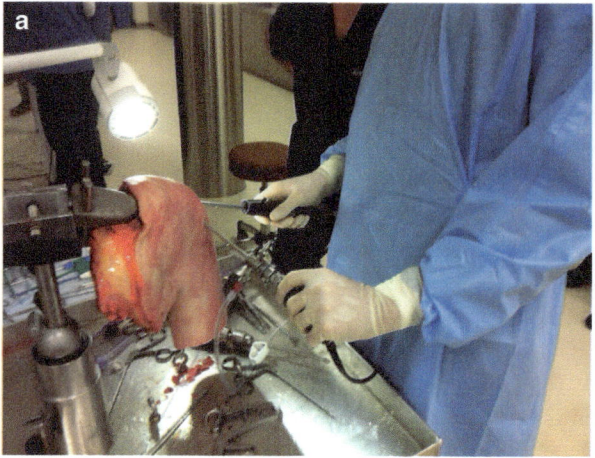
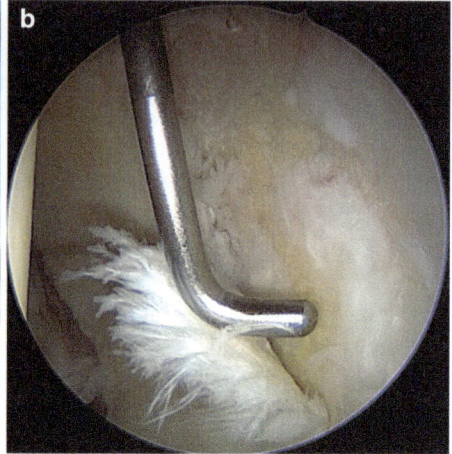

Fig. 5.8 (a) Training of acromioplasty in shoulder cadaver (© M Mayr, 2014. Reprinted with permission). (b) Arthroscopic picture of severe cartilage lesion of the acetabulum in the hip (© M Dienst, 2014. Reprinted with permission)

techniques can be trained with regard to the thick and rigid soft tissue surrounding the joint. The anterior neurovascular structures should be explored by dissection.

In elbow cadaver joints, the dorsal and radial approaches and their relation to neurovascular structures can be studied. Initially, two portals are created in the anterior part of the joint over which the joint space is inspected. Inflammation of the synovial membrane can be detected and removed. Loose bodies can also be eliminated. Restricted movement due to osteophytes and exostoses can be treated. A special feature in the joint space around the radial head can be a thickened plica humeroradialis, which clamps at movements of the joint and can cause discomfort. The dorsal approaches give access to cartilage damage, loose bodies, and adhesions in the posterior part of the elbow. Finally, the fossa olecrani can be examined and treated.

Radiocarpal joint, midcarpal joint, and distal radioulnar joint can be inspected and treated by wrist arthroscopy in cadaver joints. A special set of instruments and a special arthroscopic technique are required. Usually, smaller optical instruments are used with a diameter of 2.4 mm. Particularly useful is wrist arthroscopy for detection of damage to the cartilage and the ligament system of the wrist as well as in cases of suspected damage to the discus.

In the ankle joint, the arthroscopy approaches, diagnostic survey, retrograde drilling, microfractures, removal of loose bodies, synovectomy, osteochondral transfer, and stabilization of the syndesmosis can be trained. The challenge of the ventral and dorsal approaches can be detected. So, the surgeon is able to avoid damage to the neurovascular structures in patient treatment.

Overall, when training in different cadaver joints, arthroscopic anatomy and various joint approaches can be studied and especially in combination with post-training resection, specialized instrumentation can be handled and specific techniques can be trained.

5.4 Discussion of Cadaver Models

Although the realism is more than in plastic models and box trainers, animals are similar to cadavers in that they are expensive, they are not reusable, and there is lack of feedback (Madan and Pai 2014). Other advantages are their cost-effectiveness, easy handling, montage, and storage as well as realistic osteotomy training options compared to human cadavers. Although animal cadavers are more readily available, their usage is limited mostly due to significant anatomic differences compared to human joints.

Also, some countries have banned their use for training purposes, and maintaining an animal laboratory is expensive and requires "licensed animal caretakers, housing, veterinary care, anesthesia, and the disposal of hazardous wastes" and longer preparation times (Balcombe 2004).

The largest asset of cadaveric specimens is that they offer the most realistic simulation environment in terms of tissue appearance and sensory feedback. Per specimen, natural clinical variation is present, and tissue can be cut, drilled, or sutured similarly as in the patient. Another major advantage of using human cadavers compared to animal cadavers or other simulation means is the possibility to study exact human anatomy. Training on dry joint models has shown to support arthroscopy training on cadaver specimen but cannot replace it (Butler et al. 2013).

Also, quite some drawbacks of using cadaveric specimens for training purposes can be summed. First, they offer limited possibilities to provide feedback on performance and unpredictable the natural variation (Meyer et al. 1993). Second, the tissue may be unnaturally rigid, depending on preparation. Fresh frozen specimen are preferred as they provide realistic tissue behavior, whereas embalmed cadaver may not be sufficiently flexible (Madan and Pai 2014). Third, human cadaver teaching is restricted due to limits on availability due to local regulations and ethical guidelines (Hodgins and Veillette 2013). Often, cadavers from elderly are available which so signs of the time such as advanced osteoarthritic changes or amputated or isolated body parts are available which show an altered anatomy. The latter results in limited ability to evaluate joint anatomy with regard to surrounding muscles. Incomplete cadaver limbs result in unnatural fixation and abnormal joint stressing moments which, for example, complicates the proper dilating of the medial and lateral compartment in the knee joint. Fourth, human cadavers are expensive to purchase (between 800€ and 4,000€).

Nevertheless, cadaver courses are popular and offered by most of arthroscopic residency programs (Madan and Pai 2014). These short training courses provide a platform for novice surgeons to learn new skills and for experts to refresh the skills.

5.5   Industry Involvement

Industry involvement in orthopedic practice is an approved manner under strict regulations (Birkhahn et al. 2009). Commercial companies supporting orthopedic research supply inpatient care, and education is highly welcome in the orthopedic communities, but with academic hesitance. Industry accounts for 60 % of the financial support for clinical research and over 50 % of the funding for physician education (Birkhahn et al. 2009). Companies provide educational support to the practicing surgeon through company employee, peer to peer, printed matter (booklets, books), online materials (education platforms, surgical technique archives), company meetings (live surgery based), reserved sessions in society meetings, and time in company running cadaver labs.

Some companies have invested major sources (financial and intellectual) in human cadaver labs. We performed a questionnaire containing 16 questions among the top 8 arthroscopy industries to gain insight in their teaching programs – in alphabetical order: Arthrex, Biomet, ConMed, DePuy Synthes, Richard Wolf, Smith & Nephew, Storz, and Stryker.

The answers were processed anonymously (Table 5.1). The cadaver labs are officially run by professionals appointed by the company itself and an academic curriculum is set by company-related surgeons and assisted by staff with an educational background at six companies. Time slots are booked far in advance, which shows that education in these facilities is highly popular. Despite its high reputation and acceptance, their role in training has not been academically evaluated. "Industry, education, and arthroscopy" keywords did not retrieve any results. In order to receive the highest benefit from these facilities, a high level of collaboration is required between academia and industry.

The primary focus of the orthopedic surgeon is to improve patient care. The development of new arthroscopic technologies and equipment as well as training opportunities is provided mainly in collaboration with the industry. The industry plays an important role in the arthroscopic

Table 5.1 Inventory of industry involvement in teaching arthroscopy

Questions	Positive answers			
Does your company provide educational support to surgeons?	100 %			
Do you have a separate department for physician training?	100 %			
Does your company have a video platform?	75 %			
Does your company have an e-learning platform?	50 %			
Do you have staff with an educational background?	75 %			
Do you perform post-course evaluation?	87.5 %			
Who does the evaluation?	75 % self-evaluation			
What programs do you offer?	Clinical observation in a medical center	100 %	Live surgery sessions	100 %
	Hands-on fellowship in a medical center	37.5 %	Skill courses	100 %
For which of these joints do you offer training?	Knee	100 %	Shoulder	100 %
	Ankle	100 %	Elbow	75 %
	Hip	100 %	Wrist	75 %
How long is your course?	0.5–3 days			
In a typical educational program you offer, what is the percentage of invited consultants for teaching?	0–25 %	12.5 %	51–75 %	12.5 %
	26–50 %	63 %	76–100 %	12.5 %
What is your usual group size?	10–20 participants	50 %	31–40 participants	12.5 %
	21–30 participants	12.5 %	Depends on participant group	25 %
What percentage of theoretical lectures do you allow?	0–25 % lectures	37.5 %	Depends on the course	25 %
	26–50 % lectures	37.5 %		
Which training means do you use in your courses?	Task trainers	25 %		
	Anatomic bench models	100 %	Animal cadavers	50 %
	Virtual reality trainers	12.5 %	Human cadavers	100 %

training of residents. Visits to the clinics and accompanying surgeries by company employees are another well-established mode of educational support (Table 5.1). Educational activity performed by a surgeon who has disclosed relationship with a certain company is probably one of the most enjoyable educational settings for residents. Company-printed matters are usually neglected by the surgeons and their use is limited to support of the verbal encounter that is taking place at the time. Online material is on the increasing edge for a long while and it is expected to increase further. Obvious reasons of having immediate access at all times to any need for information are indispensable at our digital age. Company meetings that promote an exceptional surgeon in a live surgery setting to a high number of attendants are also an attractive educational environment (Table 5.1). Academic quality is expected to increase one notch if a similar setting takes place in a society meeting. Conflicts of interest should be avoided and professionalism in maintaining productive relationships with industry a goal (Poehling et al. 2008).

Bibliography

Balcombe J (2004) Medical training using simulation: toward fewer animals and safer patients. Altern Lab Anim 32(Suppl 1B):553–560, available from: PM:23581135

Birkhahn RH, Jauch E, Kramer DA, Nowak RM, Raja AS, Summers RL, Weber JE, Diercks DB (2009) A review of the federal guidelines that inform and influence relationships between physicians and industry. Acad Emerg Med 16(8):776–781, available from: PM:19594459

Butler A, Olson T, Koehler R, Nicandri G (2013) Do the skills acquired by novice surgeons using anatomic dry models transfer effectively to the task of diagnostic knee arthroscopy performed on cadaveric specimens? J Bone Joint Surg Am 95(3):e15–e18, available from: PM:23389795

Grechenig W, Fellinger M, Fankhauser F, Weiglein AH (1999) The Graz learning and training model for arthroscopic surgery. Surg Radiol Anat 21(5):347–350, available from: PM:10635100

Henn RF III, Shah N, Warner JJ, Gomoll AH (2013) Shoulder arthroscopy simulator training improves shoulder arthroscopy performance in a cadaveric model. Arthroscopy 29(6):982–985, available from: PM:23591380

Hodgins JL, Veillette C (2013) Arthroscopic proficiency: methods in evaluating competency. BMC Med Educ 13:61, available from: PM:23631421

Hui Y, Safir O, Dubrowski A, Carnahan H (2013) What skills should simulation training in arthroscopy teach residents? A focus on resident input. Int J Comput Assist Radiol Surg 8(6):945–953, available from: PM:23535939

Madan SS, Pai DR (2014) Role of simulation in arthroscopy training. Simul Healthc 9(2):127–135, available from: PM:24096921

Mattos e Dinato MC, Freitas MF, Iutaka AS (2010) A porcine model for arthroscopy. Foot Ankle Int 31(2):179–181, available from: PM:20132758

Meyer RD, Tamarapalli JR, Lemons JE (1993) Arthroscopy training using a "black box" technique. Arthroscopy 9(3):338–340, available from: PM:8323624

Morris AH, Jennings JE, Stone RG, Katz JA, Garroway RY, Hendler RC (1993) Guidelines for privileges in arthroscopic surgery. Arthroscopy 9(1):125–127, available from: PM:8442822

Patel D, Guhl JF (1983) The use of bovine knees in operative arthroscopy. Orthopedics 6(9):1119–1124, available from: PM:24822909

Pedowitz RA, Esch J, Snyder S (2002) Evaluation of a virtual reality simulator for arthroscopy skills development. Arthroscopy 18(6):E29, available from: PM:12098111

Poehling GG, Lubowitz JH, Brand R, Buckwalter JA, Wright TM, Canale ST, Cooney WP III, D'Ambrosia R, Frassica FJ, Grana WA, Heckman JD, Hensinger RN, Thompson GH, Koman LA, McCann PD, Thordarson D (2008) Patient care, professionalism, and relations with industry. Arthroscopy 24(1):4–6, available from: PM:18182194

Safir O, Dubrowski A, Mirsky L, Lin C, Backstein D, Carnahan A (2008) What skills should simulation training in arthroscopy teach residents? Int J Comput Assist Radiol Surg 3(5):433–437

Slade Shantz JA, Leiter JR, Collins JB, MacDonald PB (2013) Validation of a global assessment of arthroscopic skills in a cadaveric knee model. Arthroscopy 29(1):106–112, available from: PM:23177383

Splawski R (2011) Animal model of humeral joint for shoulder arthroscopy training. Chir Narzadow Ruchu Ortop Pol 76(6):324–326, available from: PM:22708318

Unalan PC, Akan K, Orhun H, Akgun U, Poyanli O, Baykan A, Yavuz Y, Beyzadeoglu T, Nuran R, Kocaoglu B, Topsakal N, Akman M, Karahan M (2010) A basic arthroscopy course based on motor skill training. Knee Surg Sports Traumatol Arthrosc 18(10):1395–1399, available from: PM:20012013

Vitale MA, Kleweno CP, Jacir AM, Levine WN, Bigliani LU, Ahmad CS (2007) Training resources in arthroscopic rotator cuff repair. J Bone Joint Surg Am 89(6):1393–1398, available from: PM:17545443

Voto SJ, Clark RN, Zuelzer WA (1988) Arthroscopic training using pig knee joints. Clin Orthop Relat Res 33(226):134–137, available from: PM:3335089

Wolf BR, Britton CL (2013) How orthopaedic residents perceive educational resources. Iowa Orthop J 33:185–190, available from: PM:24027481

Physical Simulators

6

Tim Horeman, Kash Akhtar,
and Gabriëlle J.M. Tuijthof

Take-Home Messages

- Box trainers and anatomic bench models by their inherent physical nature offer the great advantage of providing complete sensory feedback (i.e. visual and proprioceptive senses).
- Dexterity tests, box trainers and anatomic bench models are suitable for training arthroscopic skills provided that training tasks are adapted to the capabilities of the chosen simulator.
- Objective performance monitoring based on motion and force metrics is possible when using box trainers or anatomic bench models.

T. Horeman (✉)
Department of Biomechanical Engineering,
Delft University of Technology, Delft, The Netherlands
e-mail: t.horeman@tudelft.nl

K. Akhtar
Trauma & Orthopaedic Surgery,
Imperial College Healthcare NHS Trust, London, UK
e-mail: surgery@me.com; kasurgery@gmail.com

G.J.M. Tuijthof
Department of Biomechanical Engineering,
Delft University of Technology, Delft, The Netherlands

Department of Orthopedic Surgery,
Academic Medical Centre, Amsterdam, The Netherlands
e-mail: g.j.m.tuijthof@tudelft.nl

6.1 Definitions

All box trainers and anatomic bench models are physical by nature; that is why we propose to use the term 'physical simulators' as opposed to virtual reality simulators. Characterisation of these physical models can be intuitively performed using the level of realism (low fidelity vs. high fidelity) as criterion. The following definitions are made:

Box trainer is a physical training model that does not necessarily resembles a human joint. Thus, box trainers can literally exist of a *box*. For this reason, a box trainer is considered a low-fidelity simulator.

Anatomic bench model is a physical training model that does resemble a human joint. Other words used to describe these types of models are dummy, mannequin or phantom. Such models consist primarily of plastic elements that are shaped according to the anatomy of the intended joint. Although we realise that not all of these models have high resemblance with actual human joints when performing arthroscopy, we classify these models as high fidelity compared to the box trainers.

Additionally, the presence of sensors that register performance can be used as a second criterion to differentiate between types of models. Both box trainers and anatomic bench models can be equipped with sensors as will be illustrated.

M. Karahan et al. (eds.), *Effective Training of Arthroscopic Skills*,
DOI 10.1007/978-3-662-44943-1_6, © ESSKA 2015

6.2 History of Mechanical Simulators

Primitive forms of physical models were used for medical training for centuries before the introduction of plastic mannequins (Rosen 2008). From that point on, there have been attempts to simulate real-life experiences whenever a task has been considered too dangerous, expensive or distant in time or place to physically experience (Satava 1993). Like many technological advances, simulation has its origins in the military and aviation industries. The principle of providing flight training in a captive aircraft without actually taking off originated early in the twentieth century, with one of the earliest devices being the Sanders Teacher. The 1910 issue of Flight stated:

> the invention of a device which will enable the novice to obtain a clear conception of the workings of an aeroplane and conditions existent in the air without any risk personally or otherwise is to be welcomed (Haward 1910)

Other similar devices were created but were unsuccessful, mainly due to the unreliable and irregular nature of the wind, and so attention turned towards developing synthetic flight training devices.

The most successful flight simulator was the Link Trainer designed by Edwin Link in 1929 as a safe means of teaching new pilots how to fly and to reduce the cost of learning to fly by allowing students to learn some of the core skills on the ground (Engineers AASoM 2000). It was based on the vacuum technology used in automatic musical instruments and was seated on a series of organ bellows that would inflate or deflate to cause the trainer to bank, climb or drive. In this way, it was a mechanical device that translated physical movement of the control devices to pneumatic signals in order to move the trainer as an actual aircraft would.

The trainer was upgraded a few years later following the introduction of instrument flying to allow pilots to practise flying by using the instruments when the exterior conditions rendered it unsafe to rely on outside visual references alone. The US Army first showed interest in the Link Trainer in 1934 after a series of highly publicised air crashes occurring due to the inability of pilots to fly by instruments in poor visibility. The era of simulation-based training on the grounds of safety started to take off and the first Link Trainer for commercial use was bought by American Airlines in 1937.

We performed an inventory of available box trainers and anatomic bench models by searching literature databases (PubMed and Scopus), but also by searching Internet engines (Google and Yahoo) in an effort to be as complete as possible. We searched for the combination arthroscopy with model, trainer, phantom, dummy, mannequin, mock-up, teaching, learning, education, skill, psychomotor, dexterity, handiness and eye-hand coordination. They are presented in the following categories: box trainers, anatomic bench models per joint and models with sensors.

6.3 Box Trainers

6.3.1 Basic Psychomotor Skills

General dexterity testing products can be used by healthcare professionals, physiological researchers and human resource staffing personnel to assess the basic psychomotor skills of residents and surgeons (Kaufman et al. 1987). Several tools have been designed and manufactured that allow training-specific psychomotor skills such as reaction time, triangulation, manual dexterity and eye-hand coordination, which can be purchased at different supplies such as Lafayette Instrument Company (www.lafayetteevaluation. com), North Coast Medical (www.ncmedical. com) and ProHealthcareProducts (www.prohealthcareproducts.com) (Fig. 6.1). Unalan and coworkers have studied the prognostic nature of such basic dexterity tests for proficiency in arthroscopy and found that there is evidence (Unalan et al. 2010).

6.3.2 Dome Holder for Rotator Cuff and Labrum Repair

For training of specific surgical suture skills, a training environment is developed that consists of a transparent plastic dome (100 mm in diameter) that contains (segmented) discs with different

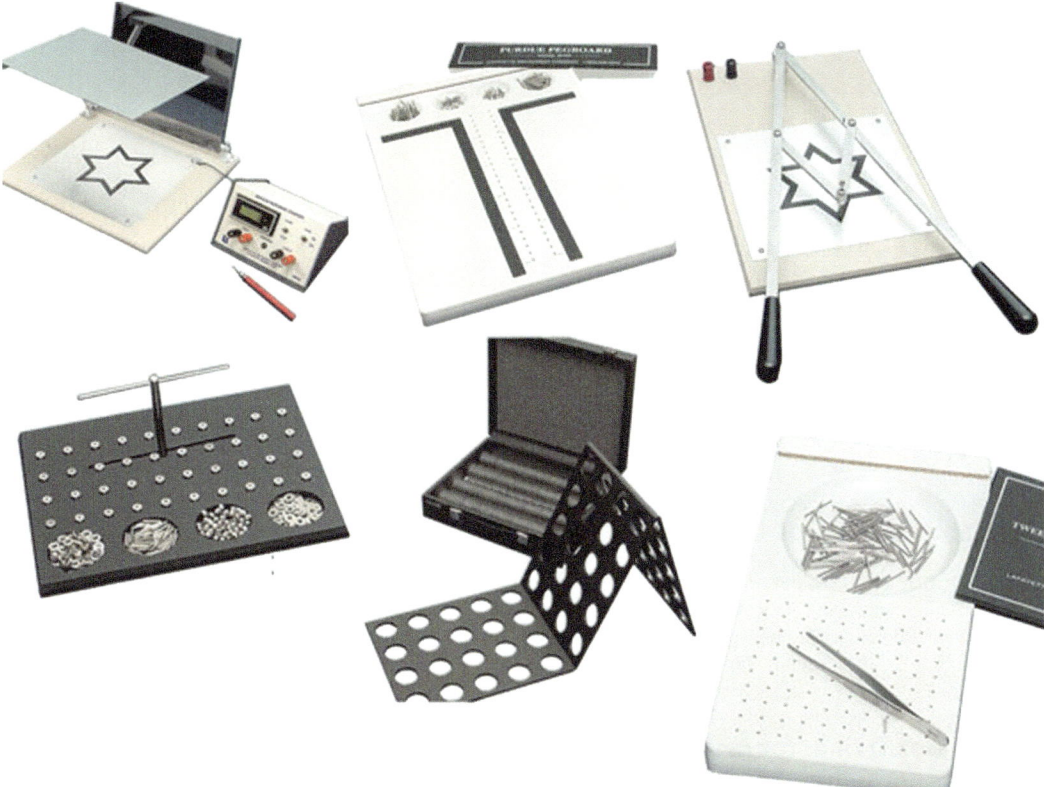

Fig. 6.1 Examples of instruments for dexterity tests. Starting in the left top corner and turning clockwise: Mirror tracer, purdue pegboard, two arm coordination tests, O'Connor Tweezer test, Minnesota manual dexterity test, Roeder manipulative aptitude test (© Lafayette Instrument Company, 2014. Reprinted with permission from www.lafayetteevaluation.com)

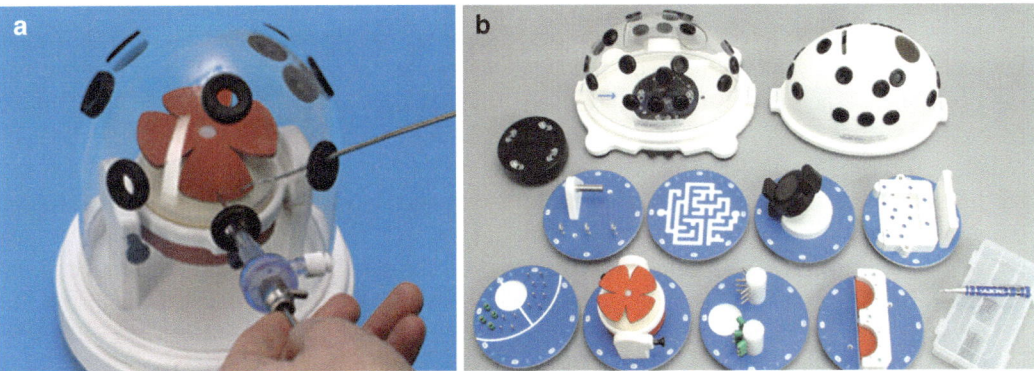

Fig. 6.2 (**a**) Dome holder for rotator cuff and labrum repair. (**b**) FAST Arthroscopy Training Workstation (© Sawbones Europe AB, 2014. Reprinted with permission from www.sawbones.com)

shapes and material densities that can be sutured (Fig. 6.2a) (www.sawbones.com). Multiple entry ports are present all around the dome to reach different locations on the disc. The discs can be locked under multiple angles to train different scenarios. The system can be used for training of standard suturing and anchor placement and be elaborated into the FAST Arthroscopy Training Workstation, involving additional basic training exercises to stimulate the psychomotor skills (Fig. 6.2b).

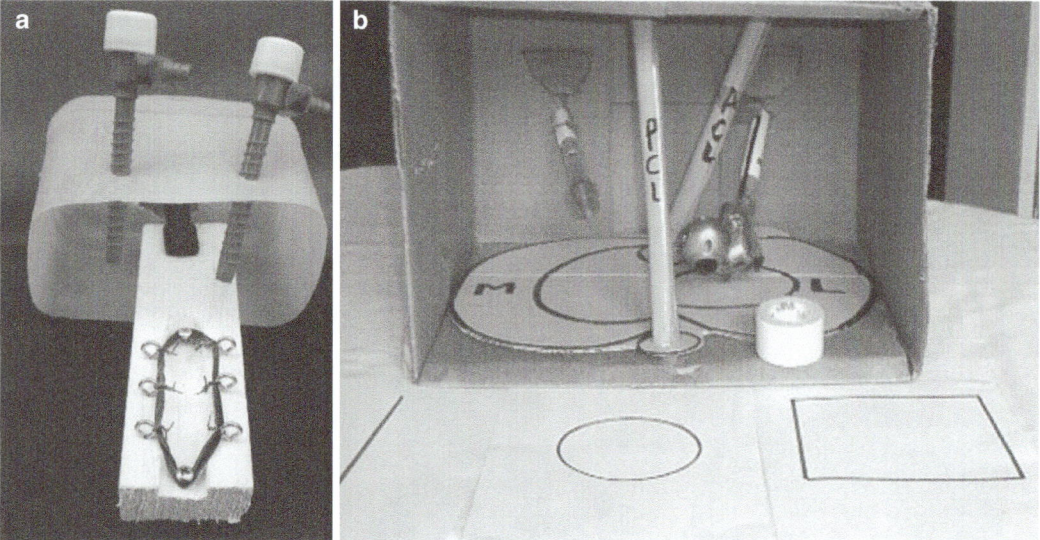

Fig. 6.3 (**a**) A model for developing psychomotor skills in arthroscopic knot tying (© Royal College of Surgeons of England, 2006. Reprinted with permission from Kitson et al. (2006)). (**b**) Simple box to train eye-hand coordination and camera positioning (© Royal College of Surgeons of England, 2009. Reprinted with permission from Patil et al. (2009))

6.3.3 Box Trainer for Arthroscopic Knot Tying

Kitson and coworkers developed a cheap and easy-to-construct jig for practising arthroscopic knot tying (Fig. 6.3a) (Kitson and Blake 2006). Six eyelets were screwed into a piece of wood with a small cut-out on one side. On each side of the eyelets, screws are placed to position two tensioned elastic bands between the two rows of eyelets. The bottom of an empty plastic container is used to simulate the tissue surrounding the entry portals and helps to fixate the trocars. While suturing the elastic band to the eyelets, a loss of suture tension during knot tying is exposed rapidly. This helps the trainee to develop psychomotor skills, to understand the concepts of sliding and locking knots and to practise a crucial step in arthroscopic shoulder surgery. This is a typical example of affordable basic psychomotor training.

6.3.4 Model for Junior Surgical Trainees

In 2009, Patil and coworkers developed a system to train bimanual camera and instrument control for arthroscopic tasks (Patil et al. 2009). A webcam was attached at 30° tilt to one end of the outer sheath of an embolectomy catheter (Fig. 6.3b). After connecting this assembly to a computer, an illuminated cardboard box was used to form an arthroscopic box trainer. A second portal in the box can be used for inserting another rod. Tasks can be performed in this box trainer aiming on bimanual coordination by contour following an instrument tip, and triangulation by manoeuvring the webcam around simulated cruciate ligaments. Although the quality of the webcam is low, the assembly is inexpensive costing around £10. Moreover, it is simple to produce and can be used repetitively with most USB cameras and computers without the necessity of operation theatre facilities. Although the authors claim that this system can hardly be a substitute for performing arthroscopy on real patients, it can improve triangulation skills and hand-eye coordination.

6.4 Anatomic Bench Models

6.4.1 Knee Joint Bench Models

This section provides an overview of the commercial knee joint bench models that to the

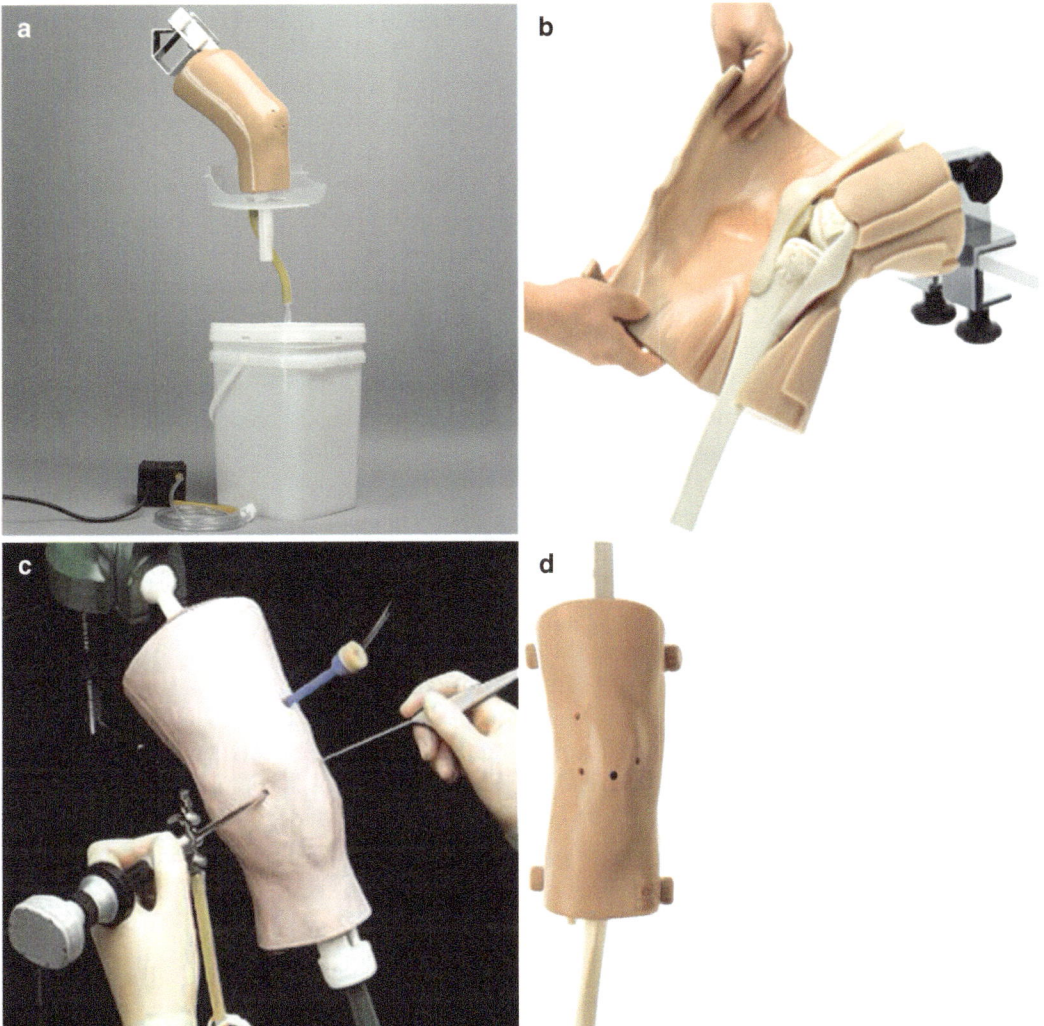

Fig. 6.4 (**a**) Sawbones knee joint bench model (© Sawbones Europe AB, 2014. Reprinted with permission from www.sawbones.com). (**b**) Adam-Rouilly knee joint bench model (© SOMSO Modelle GmbH, 2014. Reprinted with permission from www.adamrouilly.co.uk)

(**c**) Hillway Surgical Knee joint bench model (© Hillway Surgical Limited, 2014. Reprinted with permission from www.surgimodels.com). (**d**) CLA knee joint bench model (© SOMSO Modelle GmbH, 2014. Reprinted with permission from www.coburger-lehrmittelanstalt.de)

best of our knowledge are available (Fig. 6.4). For clarity, we will name them by the brand or company name. General characteristics of all knee joint bench models are that they are composed of synthetic material, equipped with a clamp to fixate the model to a solid construction and present naturally sized anatomic structures including at least skin, bones, menisci and ligaments.

Two different types of Sawbones knee joint bench models (www.sawbones.com) are available: dry or wet, which can be purchased in various sizes and can be presented on a left

or a right knee (Fig. 6.4a). Both models can be manipulated through valgus and varus and flexion and extension during training. The dry model is designed to train meniscal repair, with the menisci being replaceable. The wet model included a fluid management system and is designed to train diagnostic and operative arthroscopy techniques.

The Adam-Rouilly (www.adamrouilly.co.uk) knee joint bench model offers, beside the basic anatomic structures, also muscle and the knee joint capsule and allows removal of the cutaneous-muscular cover to show the intra-articular joint (Fig. 6.4b).

The Hillway Surgical Knee joint bench model (www.surgimodels.com) can be applied for dry and wet training. For the latter, bleedings can be simulated. The sacrificed ligaments can be replaced by new ones in a simple manner (Fig. 6.4c).

The CLA knee joint bench model (www.coburger-lehrmittelanstalt.de) has an anterior outer cover with four access points: two lateral, one central and one medial opening (Fig. 6.4d). The Hoffa's fat body is shown and can be taken off and replaced by an adhesive catch. The internal and external menisci are anchored by plug-in threads and can be easily exchanged and replaced. The cutaneous-muscular cover can be removed exposing the bones with the ligaments as a functional knee joint model.

6.4.2 Shoulder Joint Bench Models

This section provides an overview of the commercial shoulder joint bench models that to the best of our knowledge are available (Fig. 6.5). For clarity, we will name them by the brand or company name. General characteristics of all shoulder joint bench models are that they are composed of synthetic material and present naturally sized anatomic structures including at least skin, bones and ligaments.

Similarly for the knee joint models, the Sawbones shoulder bench models offer a wide variety in terms of size, left/right shoulder and dry and wet (www.sawbones.com). Figure 6.5a shows Alex III Shoulder Professor model, which has a characteristic of transparent hard-shell cover with prefabricated portals, and Fig. 6.5b shows the Arthroscopy Shoulder model covered by a soft skin that allows palpation and training of portal creation.

Internal components of the models can be replaced and allow training of various scenarios such as anchor insertion, suture passing and knot tying techniques and repair of various ligaments (SLAP, rotator cuff), tendons (biceps, subscapularis), labrum locations (posterior, anterior) and Hill-Sachs lesions.

The Hillway Surgical Shoulder joint bench model (www.surgimodels.com) can be fixated in any plane such as 'lateral decubitus' or 'beach chair' position due to multidirectional clamp.

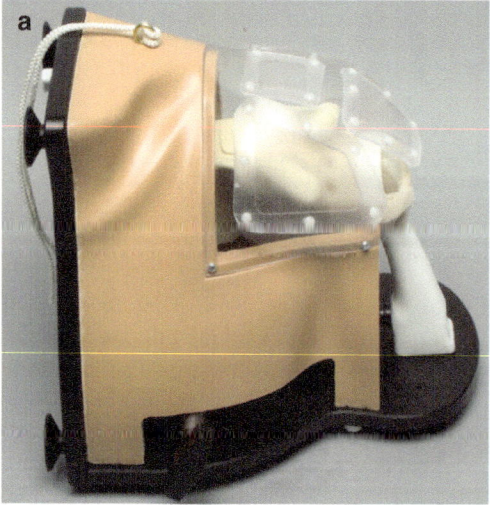
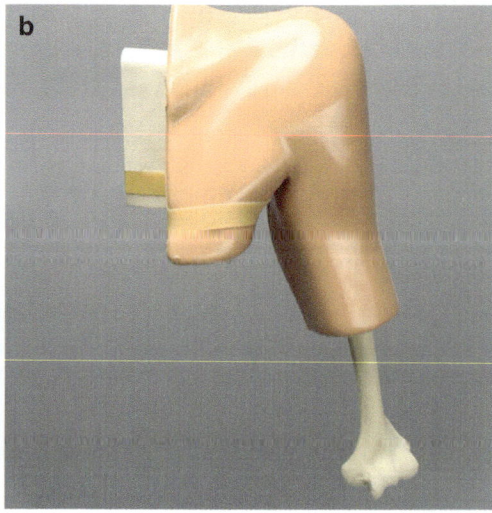

Fig. 6.5 (**a**) Sawbones Alex III Shoulder Professor model (© Sawbones Europe AB, 2014. Reprinted with permission from www.sawbones.com). (**b**) Sawbones Arthroscopy Shoulder model (© Sawbones Europe AB, 2014. Reprinted with permission from www.sawbones.com). (**c**) Hillway Surgical Shoulder joint bench model (© Hillway Surgical Limited, 2014. Reprinted with permis- sion from www.surgimodels.com). (**d**) Adam-Rouilly Shoulder joint bench model (© SOMSO Modelle GmbH, 2014. Reprinted with permission from www.adamrouilly. co.uk). (**e**) CLA shoulder joint bench model (© SOMSO Modelle GmbH, 2014. Reprinted with permission from www.coburger-lehrmittelanstalt.de). (**f**) Beijing Yimo Shoulder Joint

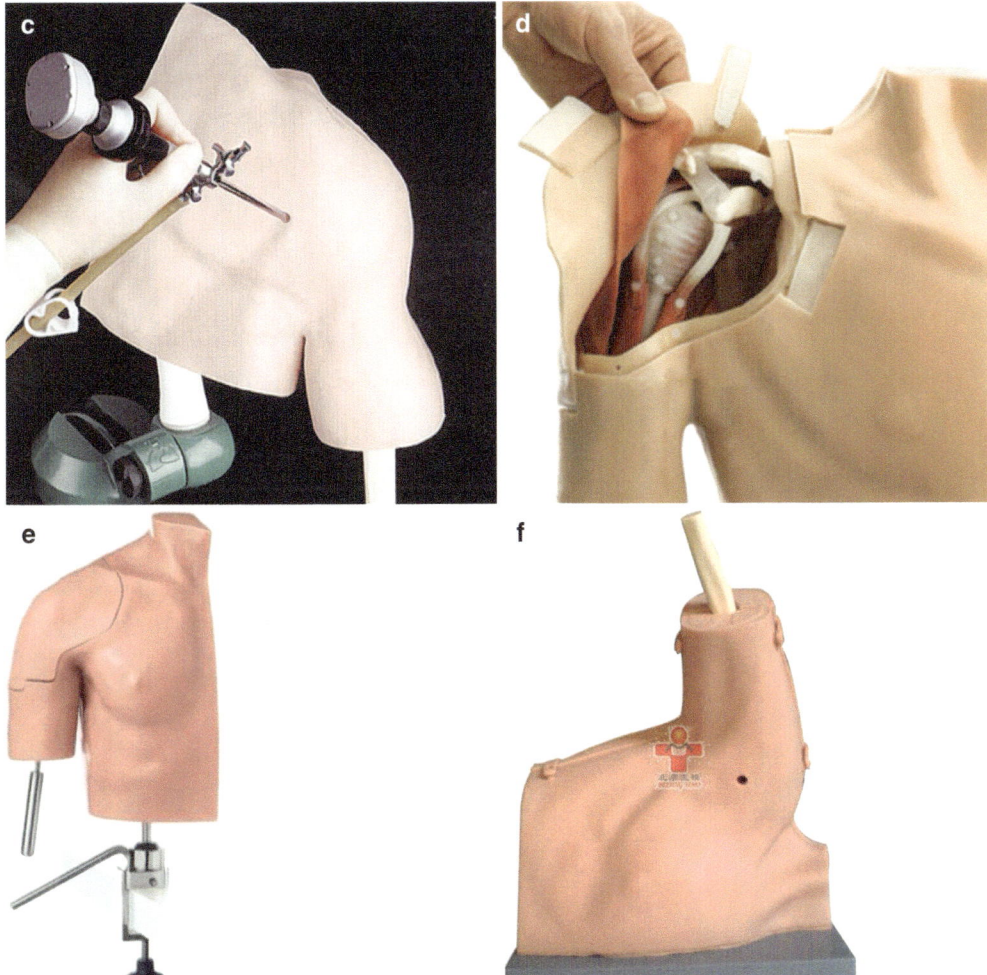

Fig. 6.5 (continued)

Removal of loose bodies, Bankart repair, labrum or biceps tendon repair and subacromial decompressions can be trained multiple times by replacing the sacrificed components with new ones (Fig. 6.5c).

The other three types of shoulder joint bench models (Adam-Rouilly Shoulder www.adamrouilly.co.uk, CLA Shoulder www.coburger-lehrmittelanstalt.de, Beijing Yimo Shoulder Joint www.chinamedevice.com) have a similar build which consist of a removable cutaneous-muscular cover to show the intra-articular joint (Fig. 6.5d–f). This allows the models to be also used as functional anatomic models during lectures. The same type of procedures as mentioned for the Sawbones models can be trained again by replacing sacrificed components.

6.4.3 Wrist Joint Bench Models

This section provides an overview of the wrist joint bench models that to the best of our knowledge are available (Fig. 6.6). If applicable, we will name them by the brand or company name. General characteristics of all wrist joint bench models are that they are composed of synthetic material and present naturally sized anatomic structures including at least skin and bones.

The Sawbones Arthroscopy Wrist Bench Model

The Sawbones Arthroscopy Wrist bench model (www.sawbones.com) is used for diagnostic techniques (Fig. 6.6a). The model contains colour-coded proximal and distal bones with volar ligaments attached.

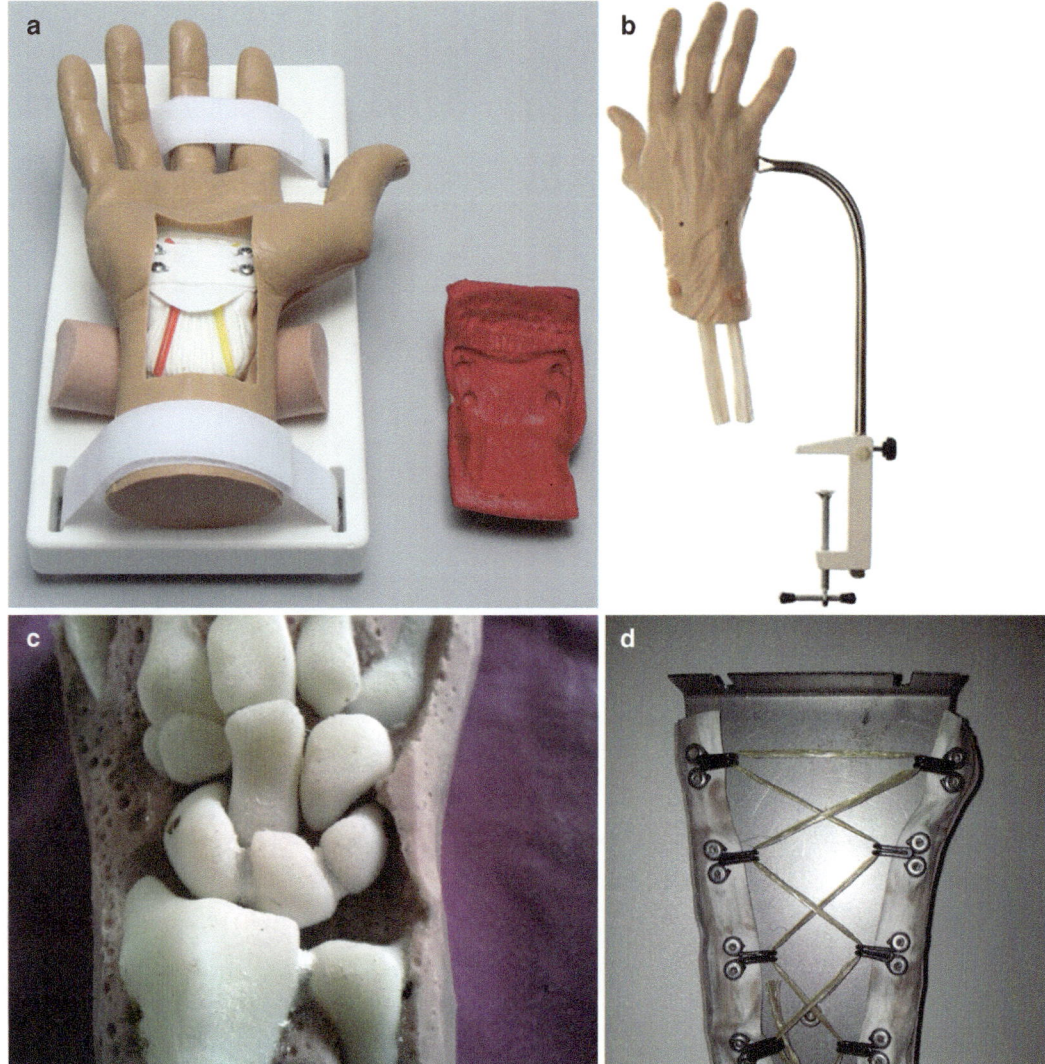

Fig. 6.6 (**a**) Sawbones Arthroscopy Wrist bench model (© Sawbones Europe AB, 2014. Reprinted with permission from www.sawbones.com) (**b**) CLA Arthroscopy Wrist bench model (Sources: websites of the companies. © SOMSO Modelle GmbH, 2014. Reprinted with permission from www.coburger-lehrmittelanstalt.de).

(**c**) Intra-articular structure AMC-TU Delft wrist model (© GJM Tuijthof, 2014. Reprinted with permission) (**d**) Special design of the skin of the AMC-TU Delft wrist model, which is placed on the back side (© GJM Tuijthof, 2014. Reprinted with permission)

The CLA Arthroscopy Wrist bench model (www.coburger-lehrmittelanstalt.de) consists of a plastic hand in which the carpal bones, the radius and ulna, together with the carpal disc and the intra-articular ligaments are visible (Fig. 6.6b). On the extensor side of the hand, two access portals are available to the inner cavity of the joint: a radiodorsal and an ulnodorsal portal. The carpal disc can be attached to the ulna and

the carpal ligaments on both the flexor and extensor sides. This structure can be exchanged or replaced as required. The model allows training for diagnosis.

One non-commercial wrist bench model is presented, which is a joint development performed by the Academic Medical Centre in Amsterdam and Delft University of Technology (Fig. 6.6c). The model is focused on training of 'portal creation' and 'navigation and identification' tasks using the arthroscope and a probe. The bony structure is a 3D print of a normal human wrist imaged with CT in distraction. To connect the carpal bones and keep them aligned while still allowing for limited movement between the bones, they were fixed in a volar plate made of silicone. Effort was put in a realistic feel of the skin and repetitive training of portal creation. Therefore, we fabricated two instead of one single skin layer. The top layer was made of silicone and 1 mm thick. The second layer was 2.5 mm consisted of silicone as well but was reinforced with medical gauze to increase tear strength. In between the silicone layers, oil was added that allows skin shifting upon palpation. The silicon material has a shore A hardness of 10, which is in the predetermined range of human skin (Kissin et al. 2006), and offers a realistic sensation of the skin. This configuration was attached around the carpal bones with a lacing system to allow adequate tensioning and quick replacement. This prototype is further developed and validated.

6.4.4   Other Joint Bench Models

Arthroscopy is performed on many more joints than the knee, the shoulder and the wrist, but to the best of our knowledge, the only company that offers anatomic bench models to train arthroscopic skills in specific other joints is Sawbones (www. sawbones.com). In Fig. 6.7, joint models of the ankle, hip and elbow are shown. They show a similar set up as presented for the other Sawbones products and provide training for the treatment of cartilage erosion of the capitellum, fracture of the radial head and loose bodies in the elbow, transcondylar fracture at various locations of the talus, chondromalacia and a osteochondral loose bodies in the ankle and labrum tears and cartilage erosion in the hip.

6.5   Models with Sensors

6.5.1   Anatomic Bench Models Combined with Sensors

For validation purposes of the use of anatomic bench models or determination of what metrics are able to discriminate between expert and novice arthroscopists, these bench models have been combined with sensor systems. We specifically use the term combine as the sensors were not physically integrated with the anatomic bench models. We provide an overview.

The most straightforward application is the use of a stopwatch to measure the completion time of a task. Scientific literature does present studies where only task time was measured, but usually the other sensors give task time as an accompanying measure when monitoring other metrics, such a motion of force metrics.

Motion metrics including path length, instrument velocity and smoothness are related to instrument or hand motion for which electromagnetic

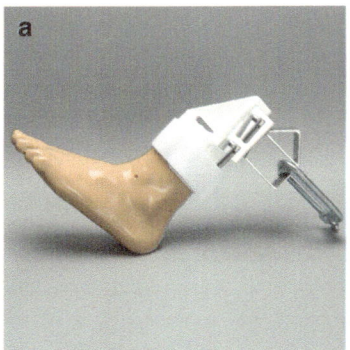
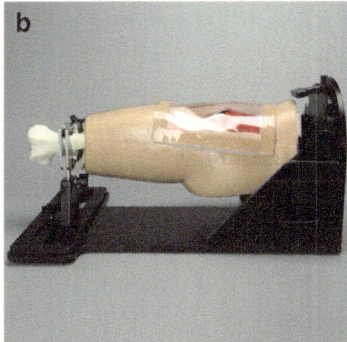
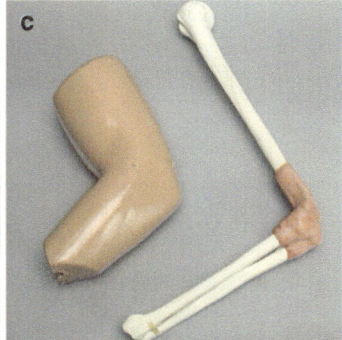

Fig. 6.7 (**a**) Sawbones ankle bench model. (**b**) Sawbones hip bench model. (**c**) Sawbones elbow bench model (© Sawbones Europe AB, 2014. Reprinted with permission from www.sawbones.com)

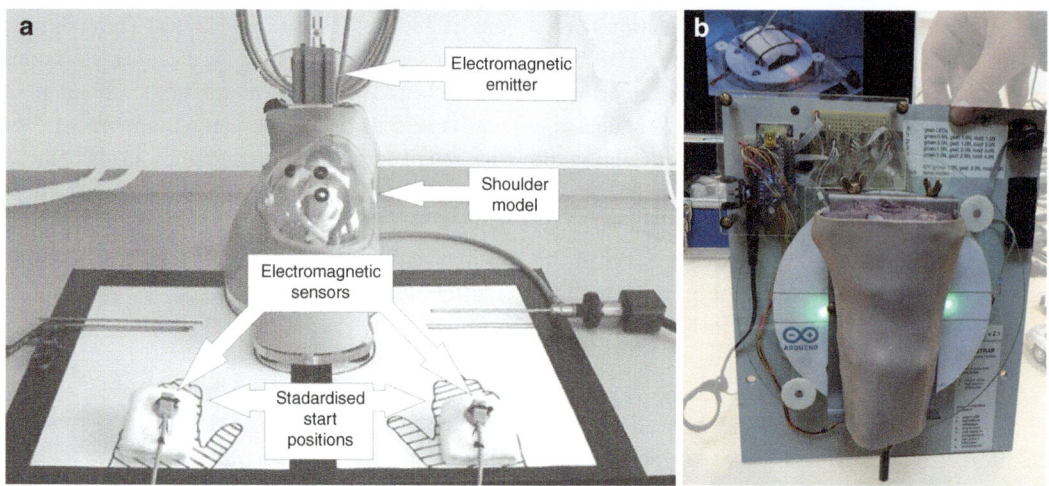

Fig. 6.8 (**a**) Alex Shoulder Professor bench top model combined with an electromagnetic motion tracking system (Reprinted from Howells et al., Copyright (2008b), with permission from Elsevier) (**b**) Force measurement system connected to the AMC-TU Delft wrist bench model (Horeman et al. 2010; © Tim Horeman, 2012. Reprinted with permission)

motion tracking systems were used (Howells et al. 2008a, 2009; Tashiro et al. 2009) (Fig. 6.8). These electromagnetic markers were attached to the instruments or the dorsum of the hands during task training on a bench model. The models that were used are the Alex Shoulder Professor (Howells et al. 2008a; Howells et al. 2009) and the knee joint bench model (Howells et al. 2008b; Tashiro et al. 2009), both from Sawbones. All four studies showed a significant difference in performance between experts and novices, and it was concluded that the motion analysis system could subsequently be used to track performance progression when practising arthroscopic skills on bench top models.

Force metrics include peak forces, average force and overall force over time. Such metrics can be determined when measuring with a six-degree-of-freedom sensor that measures the force in three directions and moments in three directions. The force sensor was attached in between the fixation table and the knee joint bench model (Tashiro et al. 2009). The results indicate that the three force metrics were also able to discriminate between experts and novices.

A similar type of 3D force sensor has been designed by Horeman and coworkers (Horeman et al. 2010) specifically for training of endoscopic skills. This platform is accurate and affordable, can be attached to various anatomic bench models and offers the possibility to record task time and all exerted forces on a computer and to provide direct feedback when manipulation forces are exceeded (Fig. 6.8b). A commercial version called ForceTRAP v2 © is available via MediShield (www.medishielddelft.com).

6.5.2   Practice Arthroscopic Surgical Skills for Perfect Operative Real-Life Treatment (PASSPORT)

The PASSPORT is a co-development project between the Academic Medical Centre in Amsterdam and Delft University of Technology (Tuijthof et al. 2010). The philosophy of PASSPORT was to combine the strong features of virtual reality systems and physical models into one design and provide sufficient clinical variation, natural visual and haptic feel and direct feedback on performance. To this end, standard arthroscopic equipment was maintained and the human knee joint was replaced by a realistic dummy in which sensors are integrated to provide feedback and registration of training

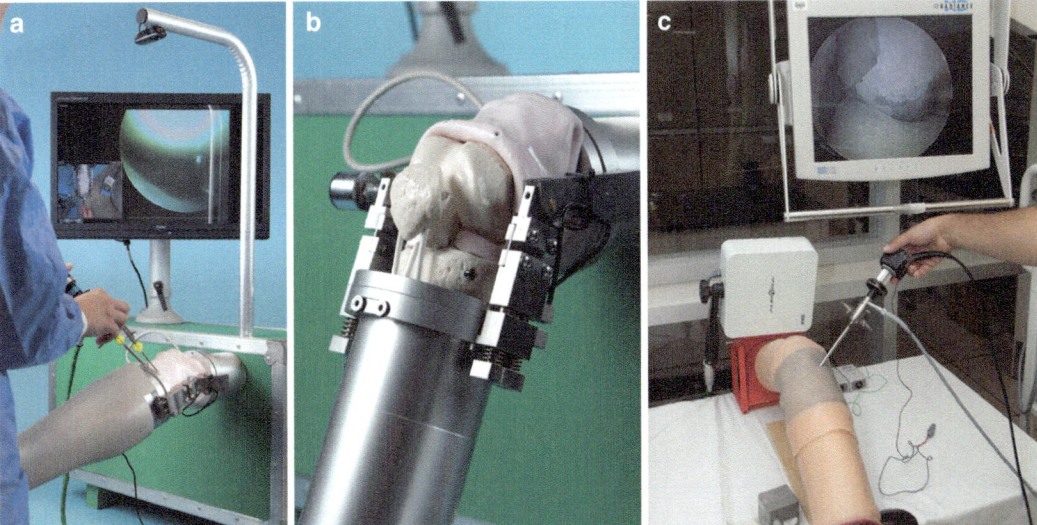

Fig. 6.9 (**a**) PASSPORT arthroscopic simulator showing the leg, instruments inserted in the joint, a webcam that tracks instrument motions and a user interface that provides the arthroscopic image and offers real-time force and time feedback during training (© AJ Loeve, 2012. Reprinted with permission). (**b**) Intra-articular joint space of PASSPORT with two forces that are connected to the tibia and femur bone to measure safe tissue manipulation (© AJ Loeve, 2012. Reprinted with permission). (**c**) Knee Arthroscopy Simulator offering motion tracking by electromagnetic sensors and allowing performance of wet arthroscopy (© 2013 IEEE. Reprinted, with permission, from Escoto et al. (2013))

sessions. After the validation of the first prototype (Tuijthof et al. 2010), PASSPORT v2 has been substantially improved (Fig. 6.9) (Escoto et al. 2013; Tuijthof and Horeman 2011; Tuijthof et al. 2012). The outer appearance of the lower leg was made from a dummy leg of a mannequin. The patella, tibia and femur bones are present, the patella moving in line with the flexion-extension motion of the lower leg. The hard plastic tibia plateau was modified for easy fixation of the menisci, which can be removed after sacrificing. This feature makes it possible to train meniscectomies and meniscus suturing. The cruciate ligaments are made of white-coloured woven rope and anatomically attached, but in such a manner that they remain in place while replacing a set of menisci. All anatomic structures match the human shape and geometry and the intra-articular joint volume was made waterproof for usage in combination with irrigation. A unique feature of PASSPORT is the special hinge that allows both flexion-extension and joint stressing in a natural manner to imitate natural knee joint stressing. Instrument motions are detected by a webcam and coloured

markers attached to the instruments, and forces exerted on the condylar femur and tibial surfaces are recorded with a special version of the 3D force sensor and directly processed for real-time feedback and performance progression (Fig. 6.9).

Similarly as when using virtual reality simulators, exercises can be designed including digital instructions and video and selection of proper metrics, as the sensors are coupled to a computer that provides a graphical user interface.

6.5.3 Knee Arthroscopy Simulator

Escoto and coworkers developed a high-fidelity knee joint bench model with performance tracking (Knee Arthroscopy Simulator) following the same line of reasoning as presented for the PASSPORT (Escoto et al. 2013). The Knee Arthroscopy Simulator is composed of modular and replaceable plastic elements which is possible with quick release clamps that uncover the intra-articular joint space (Fig. 6.9c). The lower leg is moveable and covered by a custom-made foam that holds hard plastic bones. Quick-release clamps were designed and built to tightly secure the skin surrounding the joint to the calf and the thigh, preventing water from leaking. The same electromagnetic motion tracking system as introduced above is implemented to track instrument motions, and forces are measured with a commercially available six-degree-of-freedom force sensor and by modifying the arthroscopic instruments with strain gauges. It is unclear if the simulator offers a graphical user interface that allows autonomous training.

6.6 Discussion

Dexterity tests and box trainers can be very well used to train basic psychomotor skills including eye-hand coordination, precise manipulation and bimanual tasks. Since the scientific evidence is marginal, it is recommended to extend the research with these trainers and provide additional evidence, as such tests are affordable and can be very easily translated to tests in training curricula.

Training environments in which anatomic bench models are used allow for physical interaction between the user, the instruments and the model. This immediately highlights the strong characteristic of these types of simulators: the presence of normal everyday life sensory feedback. This implies that the relevant human senses (vision and proprioception and to a lesser extend sound and smell) can be used by the trainee to acquire feedback on their performance in a natural manner. That is why anatomic bench models allow for arthroscopic therapeutic training including tissue cutting or punching and tissue reconstruction using anchors and sutures. A necessary precondition is that the simulation environment as offered by the anatomic bench models is sufficiently realistic for the intended skills training, which is so far not the case. Thus, many of these models do not present a sufficiently challenging intra-articular joint space that would allow more widespread integration of these models in the training curricula. The work done by Tuijthof and Escoto and coworkers (Escoto et al. 2013;

Tuijthof et al. 2010) indicates that engineers are aware that improvements are needed. The challenge is to keep these models affordable, which is their second biggest asset.

Both studies also indicate another disadvantage of the use of anatomic bench models, which is the lack of performance registration. This hampers individual-independent training and skill progression monitoring. Although this chapter offers several options as indicated in literature on how to combine sensors or to implement them in the anatomic bench models, most of the trainers lack a proper functioning graphical user interface that automatically processes all data and gives meaningful feedback on performance to a trainee. If physical trainers are used for educational purposes, this is definitely required for the future.

Bibliography

Engineers AASoM (2000) The link flight trainer: a historical mechanical engineering landmark. http://files.asme.org/asmeorg/Communities/History/Landmarks/5585.pdf. Accessed 31 Jan 2014

Escoto A, Le BF, Trejos AL, Naish MD, Patel RV, Lebel ME (2013) A knee arthroscopy simulator: design and validation. Conf Proc IEEE Eng Med Biol Soc 2013:5715–5718, available from: PM:24111035

Haward D (1910) The Sanders Teacher. Flight 2(50):1006–1007

Horeman T, Rodrigues SP, Jansen FW, Dankelman J, van den Dobbelsteen JJ (2010) Force measurement platform for training and assessment of laparoscopic skills. Surg Endosc 24(12):3102–3108, available from: PM:20464416

Howells NR, Brinsden MD, Gill RS, Carr AJ, Rees JL (2008a) Motion analysis: a validated method for showing skill levels in arthroscopy. Arthroscopy 24(3):335–342, available from: PM:18308187

Howells NR, Gill HS, Carr AJ, Price AJ, Rees JL (2008b) Transferring simulated arthroscopic skills to the operating theatre: a randomised blinded study. J Bone Joint Surg Br 90(4):494–499, available from: PM:18378926

Howells NR, Auplish S, Hand GC, Gill HS, Carr AJ, Rees JL (2009) Retention of arthroscopic shoulder skills learned with use of a simulator. Demonstration of a learning curve and loss of performance level after a time delay. J Bone Joint Surg Am 91(5):1207–1213, available from: PM:19411470

Kaufman HH, Wiegand RL, Tunick RH (1987) Teaching surgeons to operate – principles of psychomotor skills training. Acta Neurochir (Wien) 87(1-2):1–7, available from: PM:3314366

Kissin EY, Schiller AM, Gelbard RB, Anderson JJ, Falanga V, Simms RW, Korn JH, Merkel PA (2006)

Durometry for the assessment of skin disease in systemic sclerosis. Arthritis Rheum 55(4):603–609, available from: PM:16874783

Kitson J, Blake SM (2006) A model for developing psychomotor skills in arthroscopic knot tying. Ann R Coll Surg Engl 88(5):501–502, available from: PM:17009424

Lafayette Instrument Company (2014) Occupational skills assessment test battery. http://www.lafayette-evaluation.com/product_detail.asp?itemid=225. Accessed 28 Jan 2014

Patil V, Odak S, Chian V, Chougle A (2009) Use of webcam as arthroscopic training model for junior surgical trainees. Ann R Coll Surg Engl 91(2):161–162, available from: PM:19579297

Rosen KR (2008) The history of medical simulation. J Crit Care 23(2):157–166, available from: PM:18538206

Satava RM (1993) Virtual reality surgical simulator. The first steps. Surg Endosc 7(3):203–205, available from: PM:8503081

Stunt JJ, Kerkhoffs GM, Horeman T, van Dijk CN, Tuijthof GJM (2014) Validation of the PASSPORT V2 training environment for arthroscopic skills, Knee Surg Sports Traumatol Arthrosc, epub 8 Aug 2014 PM:25103120.

Tashiro Y, Miura H, Nakanishi Y, Okazaki K, Iwamoto Y (2009) Evaluation of skills in arthroscopic training based on trajectory and force data. Clin Orthop Relat Res 467(2):546–552, available from: PM:18791774

Tuijthof GJM, Horeman T (2011) Training facility, surgical instruments and artificial knee with an upper limb and a lower limb for simulation and training of arthroscopic surgical techniques. N2006846 (patent)

Tuijthof GJ, van Sterkenburg MN, Sierevelt IN, Van OJ, van Dijk CN, Kerkhoffs GM (2010) First validation of the PASSPORT training environment for arthroscopic skills. Knee Surg Sports Traumatol Arthrosc 18(2):218–224, available from: PM:19629441

Unalan PC, Akan K, Orhun H, Akgun U, Poyanli O, Baykan A, Yavuz Y, Beyzadeoglu T, Nuran R, Kocaoglu B, Topsakal N, Akman M, Karahan M (2010) A basic arthroscopy course based on motor skill training. Knee Surg Sports Traumatol Arthrosc 18(10):1395–1399, available from: PM:20012013

Virtual Reality Simulators

7

Kash Akhtar, Nigel J. Standfield, Chinmay M. Gupte, and Gabriëlle J.M. Tuijthof

"Nothing is as powerful as an idea whose time has come" –
Victor Hugo, Histoire d'un Crime (The History of a Crime), 1877.

Take-Home Messages
- Virtual reality knee and shoulder arthroscopy simulators allow standardized, sustained, deliberate practice.
- Virtual reality simulators can facilitate self-directed learning and let individuals progress at an appropriate pace.
- Virtual reality simulators provide accurate performance tracking and detailed feedback to inform future training and highlight areas for improvement.

K. Akhtar (✉)
Barts and the London School of Medicine and Dentistry, Queen Mary University of London, The Blizard Institute, 4 Newark Street, E1 2AT, London
e-mail: k.akhtar@qmul.ac.uk

N.J. Standfield
Department of Surgery, Imperial College Healthcare NHS Trust, London, UK
e-mail: n.standfield@imperial.ac.uk

C.M. Gupte, MRCS
Biomechanics Section, Departments of Bioengineering and Mechanical Engineering, Imperial College London, London, UK
e-mail: c.gupte@ic.ac.uk

G.J.M. Tuijthof
Department of Biomechanical Engineering, Delft University of Technology, Delft, The Netherlands

Department of Orthopedic Surgery, Academic Medical Centre, Amsterdam, The Netherlands
e-mail: g.j.m.tuijthof@tudelft.nl

7.1 Definitions

Virtual reality (VR) is defined as the computer-generated simulation of a three-dimensional image or environment that can be interacted with in a seemingly real or physical way by a person using special electronic equipment (Oxford English Dictionary 2014).

Fidelity refers to the extent to which a simulator reproduces the state and behavior of a real-world object. The more realistic it is, the higher the fidelity, and this is vital to the accurate representation of intraoperative techniques.

Haptic feedback is a method for sensory feedback that can provide a user with information regarding the contact of instruments with structures, as well as forces and possible injuries to be estimated. Haptic feedback consists of two modalities: kinesthesia and tactility.

Kinesthetic feedback, often referred to as *force feedback*, provides internal sensory information about position or movement of muscle, tendons, and bones through proprioception. Such feedback assesses both contour and stiffness of objects. Additionally, Golgi tendon organs and muscle spindles inform about applied force and opening angle of hands both applicable to arthroscopy and laparoscopy (Heijnsdijk et al. 2004).

Tactile feedback Tactility is the cutaneous perception of surface texture, pressure, heat, or pain through external contact with skin receptors. In open surgery, the surgeon relies on digital palpation to assess mechanical properties in addition

M. Karahan et al. (eds.), *Effective Training of Arthroscopic Skills,*
DOI 10.1007/978-3-662-44943-1_7, © ESSKA 2015

to temperature and the shape of tissues. Tactile feedback may discriminate between tissue states such as trauma, degenerative change, and malignancy.

7.2 History of Electronic Flight Simulators

Major technological advances occurred during World War II (WWII), coupled with the development of analog computers, meaning that the technology now existed to calculate the flight equations necessary to simulate the response to aerodynamic forces rather than the mere physical representation of their effects. Approximately 10,000 simulators were used during WWII to train more than 500,000 pilots before proceeding to actual flight training or to fine-tune the skills of experienced pilots. Interestingly, the majority of German Luftwaffe bomber pilots would also have spent a minimum of 50 h in a Link Trainer (Chap. 6).

As technology advanced, the Curtiss-Wright Corporation was contracted by Pan American Airways to construct the first full aircraft simulator for the Boeing 377 Stratocruiser in 1943. Other airlines went on to purchase similar machines, but simulator evolution began to plateau over the next decade as it became clear that analog computers could not provide the desired fidelity or reliability.

7.3 History of Digital Simulators

These obstacles were overcome by the introduction of digital computers in the 1960s and 1970s. Concomitantly, motion systems were developed to provide six degrees of freedom. NASA undertook significant research into motion systems and created a Lunar Module simulator (a larger and more complex version of the original Link Trainer) to prepare for the first moon landing of 1969. When Buzz Aldrin piloted the Lunar Module down onto the surface of the moon, he said: "*Everything is A-OK. It throttles down better than the simulator.*" The Apollo 11 crew had spent over 600 h in simulator training and the astronauts of the Apollo program had averaged approximately 936 h of simulator time each.

There was also a need for systems to provide *out-of-window* visual scenes in order to improve fidelity. The first computer-generated image (CGI) simulation systems were produced by the General Electric Company for the space program. Progress was rapid and closely linked to developments in digital computer hardware. The quality and content of the image display improved so significantly that it became possible for pilots to become familiar with routes through using the simulator. The International Air Transport Association (IATA) formed a Flight Simulator Technical Sub-Committee (FSTSC) in 1973 and set about developing the standards for simulation, and this allowed simulation to become a compulsory requirement for accreditation and completed the transfer of training and aircrew certification from the aircraft to the simulator.

Aircraft simulators nowadays typically cost between £20 and 30 million and are used 22 h a day with 2 h of downtime for maintenance. Pilots learning to fly a new aircraft typically undergo 2 weeks of *ground school* followed by 3–4 weeks of simulator training. The use of simulation has resulted in a decrease in the requirements for actual training hours on airplanes. Once accredited, pilots undergo simulator-based testing twice a year in order to maintain their licenses.

7.4 VR Simulation in Medicine

The aviation industry's experience with simulation dates back almost a century, and its success has resulted from the establishment of standards for data, design, modeling, performance, and testing, with international agreements for accreditation at defined levels of fidelity (Riley 2008). VR simulation in medicine has developed over the past two decades now in response to working hour restrictions for doctors, rising medicolegal compensation payments, and increasing focus on patient safety (McGovern 1994; Satava 1993, 1994). There is no substitute for sustained, deliberate practice. Without this there are problems with the retention of recently learned skills, and the longer the period they are not used, the greater the rate of decay (Kneebone et al. 2004). Simulation may then offer opportunities to support learning by allowing the practice and consolidation of clinical skills. There is growing evidence for simulation to be included as part of the surgical training curriculum, and it is recognized as a valuable means of practicing and improving laparoscopic skills (Aggarwal et al. 2007, 2008).

Many studies have been confined to the virtual world, but further work has shown that the effects of simulation-based training can cross over into the "real world." The use of a VR simulation-based curriculum has been shown to shorten the learning curve on laparoscopic procedures in the operating theatre (Aggarwal et al. 2008). Skills attained using the simulator can significantly improve performance in the *live* procedure (Seymour et al. 2002).

7.5   VR Simulation in Arthroscopy

The majority of orthopedic surgical procedures involve open surgery with complex anatomical and patient positioning factors that are not easily amenable to simulation. Arthroscopic procedures better lend themselves to simulation, with the conversion of three dimensions to a 2D screen easier replicated. As computer processing power has rapidly developed, the quality of graphics has facilitated realistic representations of arthroscopic procedures. The fidelity is further heightened by the use of instruments being used at a distance from the surgeon, out of the direct field of view.

Virtual reality simulators have developed as a means of addressing these issues. They have been used increasingly with time as they allow training in a safe, protected environment. Once trainees have been shown how to use the simulator, they can undertake training at their own pace at a time of their choice to achieve personal goals (Michelson 2006).

The first arthroscopic VR simulator was described in Germany in 1995 as a result of a collaboration between traumatologists and computer graphics scientists (Ziegler et al. 1995). In 1996 the American Academy of Orthopedic Surgeons (AAOS) evaluated VR technology as a means of learning and maintaining surgical skills and felt that it was too early to commit the substantial resources required (Mabrey et al. 2000; Poss et al. 2000). However, the following year, the American Board of Orthopedic Surgery (ABOS) funded the development of a prototype VR knee simulator with three aims:

- That it be embraced by the entire orthopedic community
- That the tool must be valid and reliable
- That surgeons must have experience with the simulator and have confidence that it is a realistic and useful surrogate for actual operative surgery

After this, other computer science groups from all over the world have taken initiatives to design virtual reality environments of the knee (Gibson et al. 1997; Heng et al. 2004, 2006; Hollands and Trowbridge 1996; Megali et al. 2002; Ward et al. 1998) by the application of volume rendering techniques (Gibson et al. 1997), object deformation modeling techniques for collision detection (Sherman et al. 1999, 2001; Ward et al. 1998), and computer graphics techniques to guide a trainer through exercises (Megali et al. 2002, 2005). All these initiatives have not let to commercialization.

Generally, VR arthroscopy simulators comprise a computer and screen which present the virtual world. The instruments are designed to recreate the look, feel, and/or functionality of those used in the operating theatre. These physical devices are represented on the screen and thus can be used to interact with the virtual environment. Instruments that can be recreated include cameras, probes, punches, chondral picks, and shavers. The visual graphics used by VR simulators have improved exponentially as computing power has developed, but also key is the feeling of touch, and knowing where the structure at the end of the probe is soft or hard plays an important role. That is why in general VR simulators also have a synthetic shoulder or knee joint model that can be manipulated and into which instruments can be inserted through predefined portals. These instruments can be used to manipulate virtual tissues and organs, and there may be visual feedback through the visible deformity of tissues or force feedback through a haptic device.

In minimally invasive surgery, instruments connect the hands with the tissues and act as the conduits for conveying information about the nature of intra-articular structures. Insufficient visual detail can lead to misidentification of anatomy and the increased likelihood of adverse events (Zhou et al. 2008). In the remainder of this section, several VR simulators are discussed that reflect the overall development and availability of arthroscopic VR simulators.

7.6 SKATS VR Simulator

Haptic feedback can be active or passive. The Sheffield Knee Arthroscopy Training System (SKATS) was initially designed as a cost-effective PC-based knee arthroscopy simulator consisting of a hollow plastic leg, replica surgical instruments, and a monitor displaying the internal view of the knee joint (McCarthy et al. 2006; McCarthy and Hollands 1998). A 3D computer-generated environment provided a real-time, interactive simulation of the tissue with the screen responding to the user as bimanual arthroscopic tasks are performed and the visual image is changed correspondingly. Research has shown that the effectiveness of a simulator is based on visual, haptic, and proprioceptive information. Evaluation of the original system by surgeons demonstrated severe acceptability issues as the instruments would pass through solid structures, and this is likely to affect skill acquisition and disrupt the level of immersion in the task due to the lack of reality (Moody et al. 2003).

Arthroscopy is a bimanual task that uses haptic cues for a range of tasks, and adding this to this machine would require two four-degree-of-freedom haptic devices to apply reactionary forces in response to contact with a variety of

knee structures and yet still fit within a fully manipulable physical limb model. It was therefore decided to develop this further by adding passive haptics (tactile augmentation) (Moody et al. 2008). A more realistic leg was used containing solid femur and tibia to create a mixed reality environment where physical contact is felt when touching the bone.

The validation results obtained when passive haptic feedback (resistance provided by physical structures) was provided indicate that the SKATS had construct, predictive, and face validity for navigation and triangulation training. Feedback from questionnaires completed by orthopedic surgeons indicated that the system had face validity for its remit of basic arthroscopic training. There was a desire to include haptic feedback, though a formal task analysis demonstrated that many of the core skills for trainees to learn when navigating a knee arthroscopically did not require active haptics and though the feedback highlighted the need for the menisci and ligaments to provide haptic feedback in addition to the bone. Further development of the SKATS ceased in 2004, and this system was not produced for sale.

7.7 SIMENDO Arthroscopy™

The SIMENDO Arthroscopy™ (Simendo, Rotterdam, the Netherlands, www.simendo.eu) is one of the few arthroscopic VR simulators that solely focuses on training of eye-hand coordination. The system consists of a Notebook computer and a console with three devices: a camera, a probe, and a foot with part of the lower leg (Fig. 7.1). The focus on eye-coordination training is prominently expressed in their exercises *4 Boxes* and *6 Boxes*, which take place in an entirely virtual world that does not represent a human joint and focuses solely on correct camera orientation. The VR simulator does not provide any active haptic device, so trainees rely solely on their visual feedback. Target users are residents that have no arthroscopic experience. The simulator can also be connected to the Internet, where training progress is documented and can be viewed by supervising surgeons.

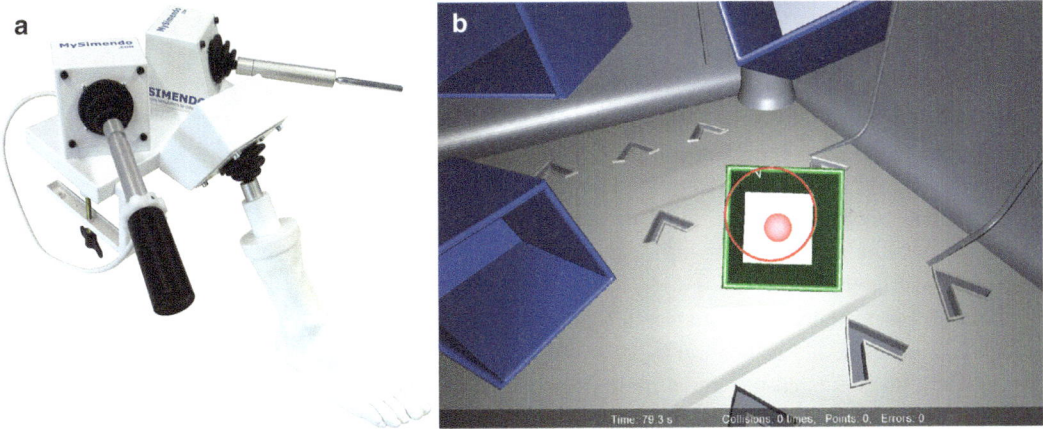

Fig. 7.1 (**a**) SIMENDO Arthroscopy™ simulator. (**b**) Screenshot from the virtual world of the *Boxes* exercises. The ball in a box needs to be touched with the camera tip (© Simendo, 2014. Reprinted with permission from www.simendo.eu)

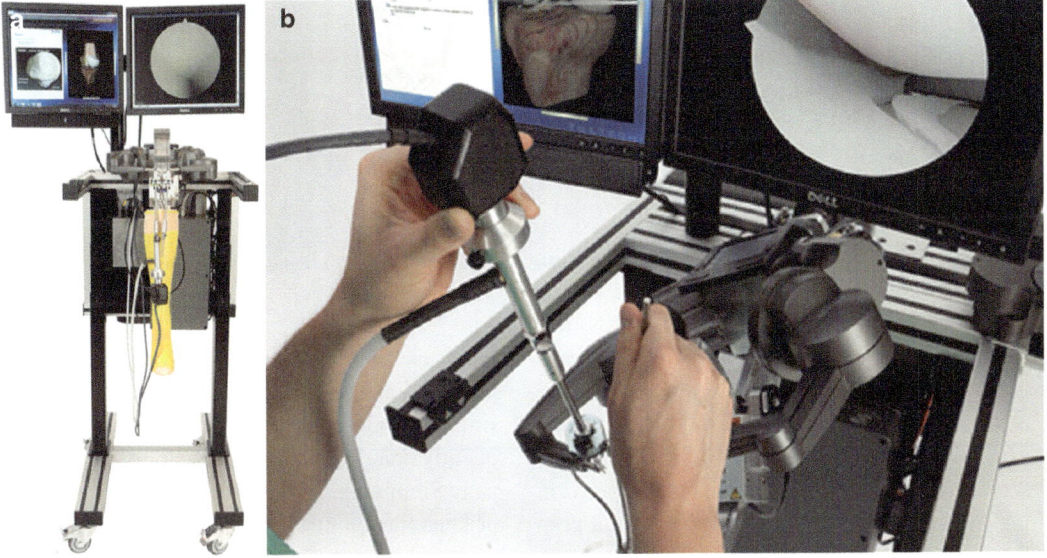

Fig. 7.2 (**a**) The Knee Arthroscopy Surgical Trainer (KAST) named ArthroSim™. (**b**) Close up of the ArthroSim controls with the arthroscope in the left hand and the probe in the right

7.8   Knee Arthroscopy Surgical Trainer: ArthroSim™

The Knee Arthroscopy Surgical Trainer (KAST) was developed by the AAOS Virtual Reality Task Force in collaboration between the ABOS, the Arthroscopy Association of North America (AANA), and Touch of Life Technologies (ToLTech, Colorado, USA, www.toltech.net) (Fig. 7.2).This platform was subsequently developed to add shoulder arthroscopy and has been renamed the ArthroSim™ Arthroscopy Simulator. This machine uses data from the Visible Human Project and has a computer hardware component supported by proprietary software and a didactic component delivered on one of two monitors positioned in front of the trainee. The core of the hardware component is a pair of high-fidelity active haptic devices (Geomagic Touch, North Carolina, USA [formerly Sensable Phantom Omni]) that monitor the position of the instruments to recreate the feel of the arthroscope and the probe within the knee.

The software represents and replicates the visual, mechanical, and behavioral aspects of the knee while task-oriented programs monitor and record performance metrics. This includes moderating the haptic interface and simultaneously executing a collision detection algorithm that prevents the instruments from moving through solid surfaces. The two-hand haptic device provides 4 degrees of freedom (DOF). The first three DOFs with force feedback consist of pitch, yaw, and insertion that enable the instrument to move in a way similar to a real arthroscope. The fourth rotational DOF is without force feedback to enable surgeons to look around the immediate vicinity of the 30° arthroscope tip, and there is also force feedback when there is a collision or when handling soft tissues.

There is a dual monitor system where the right screen displays the intra-articular image and the left screen displays the "Mentor." This provides a training program based on a curriculum developed by the AAOS. It uses movies, images, animations, and texts to outline the steps of each procedure. Trainees must achieve proficiency and score 100 % in each step before finally performing the entire procedure unaided within a community standard time.

However, the ArthroSim^{TM} is currently limited to diagnostic procedures only though there are plans to develop therapeutic tasks. It is currently undergoing validation studies at eight orthopedic residency programs in the USA and the results are awaited.

7.9   ARTHRO Mentor^{TM}

The ARTHRO Mentor^{TM} (Simbionix, Cleveland, Ohio USA, www.simbionix.com) uses the same pair of Geomagic Touch haptic devices for active

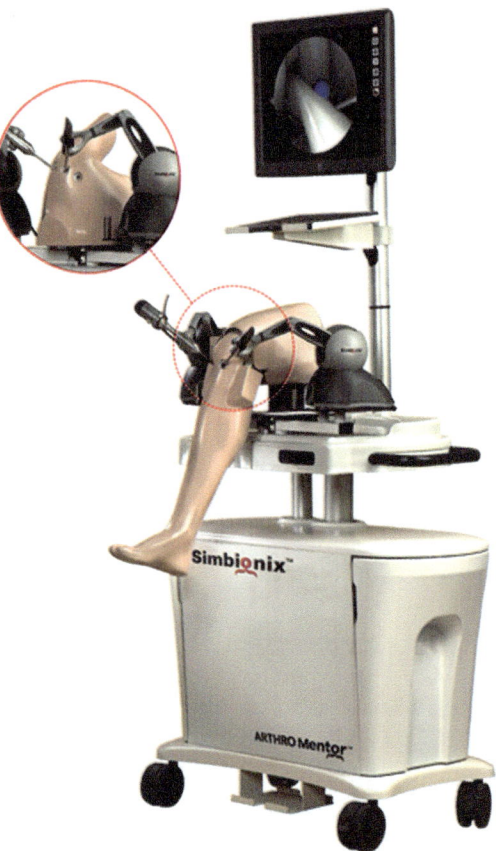

Fig. 7.3 ARTHRO Mentor^{TM} VR simulator for knee and shoulder arthroscopy

feedback (Fig. 7.3). It was initially created and marketed as the Insight ArthroVR^{TM} arthroscopy simulator (GMV, Madrid, Spain) but was subsequently bought and further developed by the company Simbionix. It consists of a synthetic shoulder or knee model attached to a platform incorporating two haptic devices, a computer and screen.

The ARTHRO Mentor^{TM} provides a sequence of training modules to help trainees develop the necessary skills to perform arthroscopic surgery. It focuses on the identification of anatomical structures, navigation skills, triangulation and depth perception, and instrument handling skills. It displays both healthy and pathological states and incorporates diagnostic and therapeutic procedures for the shoulder and knee. Similar to the other available simulators, it provides detailed and exportable feedback reports covering the distance covered by the camera and instruments, time taken, and the smoothness and efficiency of movements. Feedback is one area where VR simulators excel, and immediate visual feedback of multiple performance metrics highlights their educational potential (Howells et al. 2008b). Trainees can closely monitor their performance through variables such as time taken, path length, and number of hand movements. These metrics have been proven to correlate with surgical proficiency and thus provide valuable feedback (Datta et al. 2001; Howells et al. 2008a).

All of the commercially available highlighted simulators allow trainees to be provided with individualized and customizable learning programs. The ARTHRO Mentor is linked to *MentorLearn*, a Web-based simulator management program to help facilitate this.

7.10 VirtaMed ArthroS™ Simulator for Knee and Shoulder Arthroscopy

A new commercially available arthroscopy simulator has recently come to the market that is also centered on passive haptics (Fig. 7.4).

The VirtaMed ArthroS™ for knee and shoulder arthroscopy (VirtaMed AG, Zurich, Switzerland, www.virtamed.com) is the only available VR simulator to use a modified actual arthroscope and modified authentic instruments in order to add to fidelity and allow trainees to familiarize themselves with the equipment. It also has inlet and outlet valves for fluid handling and replicates the poor view that is encountered when this is not managed appropriately. Cameras with 0, 30, and 70° are provided, along with a probe, grasper, punch, and shaver. A synthetic knee or shoulder model is added, and the knee can be subjected to varus and valgus stresses to open up the joint compartments as required, and the shoulder model can be placed in a lateral decubitus or beach chair position.

Didactic tutorials allow trainees to use the machine independently and facilitate self-directed learning. There are guided modules for learning basic skills, modules for diagnostic arthroscopy requiring use of the probe, and modules for therapeutic arthroscopy requiring the use of the grasper, punch, or shaver.

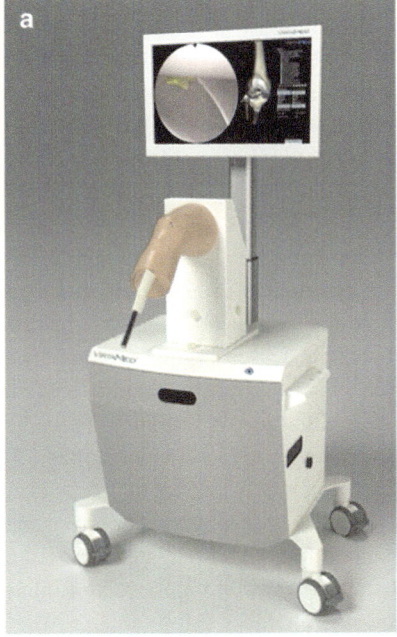
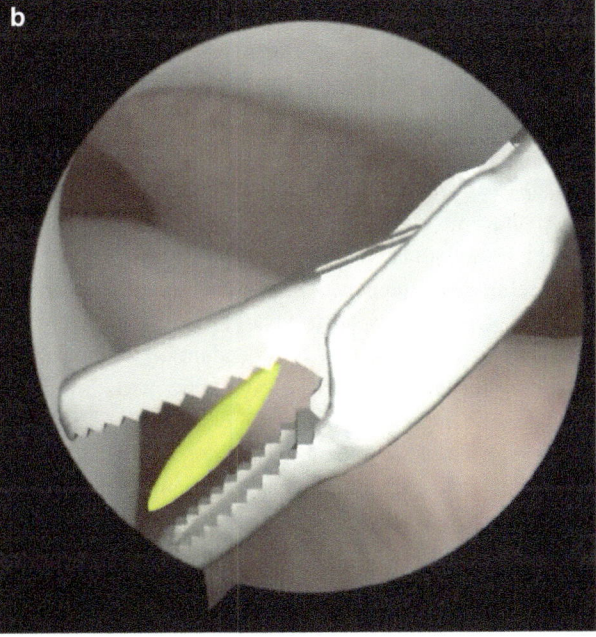

Fig. 7.4 (**a**) VirtaMed ArthroS™ for knee arthroscopy. (**b**) Training exercise using the VirtaMed ArthroS™ for knee arthroscopy. (**c**) VirtaMed ArthroS™ for shoulder arthroscopy. (**d**) Removal of loose bodies on the VirtaMed ArthroS™ for shoulder arthroscopy

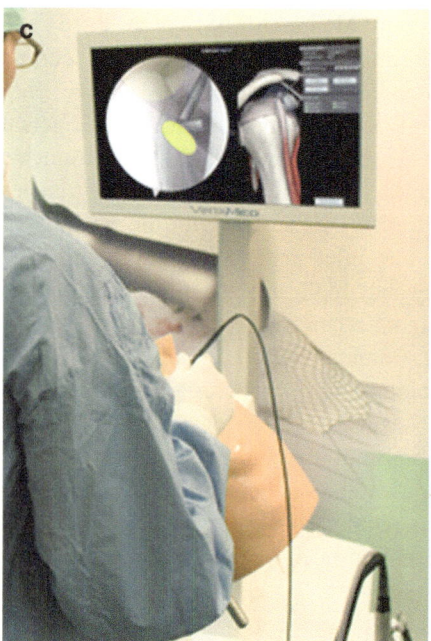
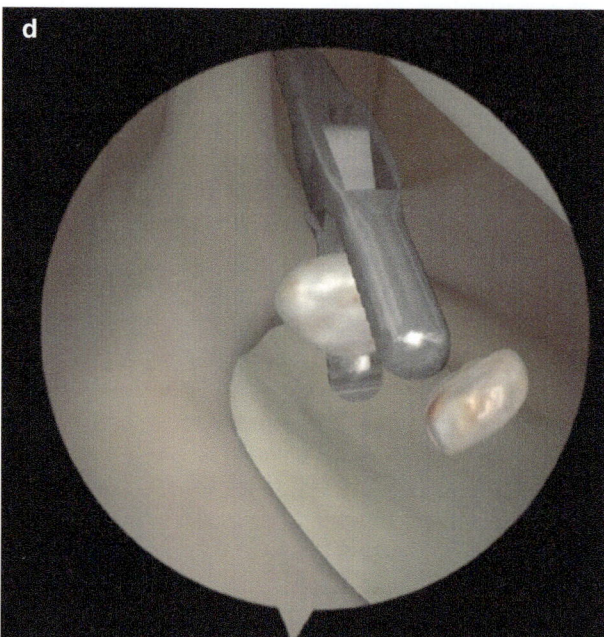

Fig. 7.4 (continued)

7.11 Discussion

VR arthroscopy simulators have repeatedly been shown to be acceptable, realistic, and effective at subjectively distinguishing between individuals of different levels of clinical experience and skill. Training on a simulator results in significant improvement in arthroscopic skills, and individuals who continue with their clinical training improve concomitantly in their simulator performance. VR simulators avoid the ethical and storage issues associated with cadavers. Cadavers require high maintenance, are not readily available, and can only be used a limited number of times, and the quality is dependent on the embalming technique employed. Synthetic models meanwhile are not reusable, can oversimplify the task, can cause significant mess, are resource and staff intensive, and have low face validity. While some VR simulators can be expensive and require periodic maintenance, this can often be done remotely online. They can be used repeatedly with no consumable parts and require less human resources. They are also compact and do not take up a significant amount of space. They can display a range of pathology and have no ethical constraints. VR simulators allow standardized, repeated practice that has high validity and reliability. They are more appropriate to self-directed learning, and trainees can progress at their own pace and at a time of their choice to achieve personal goals without the need for a senior surgeon to be present, unlike other forms of simulation-based training (Michelson 2006).

However, the current VR simulators are not without their limitations. One criticism of VR simulators has been the lack of realistic tissue behavior (Dankelman 2007). Surgeons value haptics in surgical simulators, and this has been addressed to some degree by improvement in collision detection and improved haptic feedback. This was seen with the (discontinued) Procedicus Virtual Arthroscopy trainer (Mentice Inc., San Diego, USA) which provided haptic feedback and was rated highly by participants because it made the experience of shoulder and knee procedures more realistic and showed high levels of internal consistency and reliability (Modi et al. 2010).

VR simulators are most appropriate for trainees needing to practice basic arthroscopic tasks and do not faithfully simulate the more complex tasks. There is little published research on the current commercially available simulators and there has not been any evidence of the ability of VR simulator-based training to improve arthroscopic performance in the operating theatre. Further crossover studies are needed with longitudinal follow-up of trainees undergoing VR simulation-based training to fully understand the benefits to patients. It is accepted though that simulator training can shorten the time it takes for trainees to acquire basic skills in theatre, and this has universal advantages, for trainees, trainers, institutions, and, most importantly, patients. The use of VR simulation can be an effective way for junior orthopedic trainees to quickly attain the basic technical skills specific to orthopedic surgery. Simulation-based training can cause a "right shift" along the learning curve for more efficient training with real-world improvements (Ahlberg et al. 2007; Larsen et al. 2009; Seymour et al. 2002).

In recent years, there has been a drive to integrate simulation into surgical training programs and an understanding of the need to develop validated curricula (Aggarwal et al. 2004). It has been shown that simulators can be used to create a graduated laparoscopic training curriculum and this work has been extended to create an evidence-based virtual reality training program for novice laparoscopic surgeons (Aggarwal et al. 2006a, b).

There is growing evidence for simulation to be formally integrated into the orthopedic curriculum. It should however be placed in the context of traditional training methods and regarded as a means rather than an end in itself.

Bibliography

Aggarwal R, Moorthy K, Darzi A (2004) Laparoscopic skills training and assessment. Br J Surg 91(12):1549–1558, available from: PM:15547882

Aggarwal R, Grantcharov T, Moorthy K, Hance J, Darzi A (2006a) A competency-based virtual reality training curriculum for the acquisition of laparoscopic psychomotor skill. Am J Surg 191(1):128–133, available from: PM:16399123

Aggarwal R, Grantcharov TP, Eriksen JR, Blirup D, Kristiansen VB, Funch-Jensen P, Darzi A (2006b) An evidence-based virtual reality training program for novice laparoscopic surgeons. Ann Surg 244(2):310–314, available from: PM:16858196

Aggarwal R, Ward J, Balasundaram I, Sains P, Athanasiou T, Darzi A (2007) Proving the effectiveness of virtual reality simulation for training in laparoscopic surgery. Ann Surg 246(5):771–779, available from: PM:17968168

Aggarwal R, Balasundaram I, Darzi A (2008) Training opportunities and the role of virtual reality simulation in acquisition of basic laparoscopic skills. J Surg Res 145(1):80–86, available from: PM:17936796

Ahlberg G, Enochsson L, Gallagher AG, Hedman L, Hogman C, McClusky DA III, Ramel S, Smith CD, Arvidsson D (2007) Proficiency-based virtual reality training significantly reduces the error rate for residents during their first 10 laparoscopic cholecystectomies. Am J Surg 193(6):797–804, available from: PM:17512301

Dankelman J (2007) Surgical simulator design and development. World J Surg 32(2):149–155, available from: PM:17653587

Datta V, Mackay S, Mandalia M, Darzi A (2001) The use of electromagnetic motion tracking analysis to objectively measure open surgical skill in the laboratory-based model. J Am Coll Surg 193(5):479–485, available from: PM:11708503

Gibson S, Samosky J, Mor A, Fyock C, Grimson E, Kanade T, Kikinis R, Lauer H, McKenzie N, Nakajima S, Ohkami H, Osborne R, Sawada A (1997) Simulating arthroscopic knee surgery using volumetric object representations, real time volume rendering en haptic feedback, Proceedings of CVRMed-MRCAS, pp 369–378

Heijnsdijk EA, Pasdeloup A, van der Pijl AJ, Dankelman J, Gouma DJ (2004) The influence of force feedback and visual feedback in grasping tissue laparoscopically. Surg Endosc 18(6):980–985, available from: PM:15108104

Heng PA, Cheng CY, Wong TT, Xu Y, Chui YP, Chan KM, Tso SK (2004) A virtual-reality training system for knee arthroscopic surgery. IEEE Trans Inf Technol Biomed 8(2):217–227, available from: PM:15217267

Heng PA, Cheng CY, Wong TT, Wu W, Xu Y, Xie Y, Chui YP, Chan KM, Leung KS (2006) Virtual reality techniques. Application to anatomic visualization and orthopaedics training. Clin Orthop Relat Res 442:5–12, available from: PM:16394732

Hollands R, Trowbridge E (1996) A virtual reality training tool for the arthroscopic treatment of knee disabilities, Maidenhead, pp 131–139

Howells NR, Brinsden MD, Gill RS, Carr AJ, Rees JL (2008a) Motion analysis: a validated method for showing skill levels in arthroscopy. Arthroscopy 24(3):335–342, available from: PM:18308187

Howells NR, Gill HS, Carr AJ, Price AJ, Rees JL (2008b) Transferring simulated arthroscopic skills to the operating theatre: a randomised blinded study. J Bone Joint Surg Br 90(4):494–499, available from: PM:18378926

Kneebone RL, Scott W, Darzi A, Horrocks M (2004) Simulation and clinical practice: strengthening the relationship. Med Educ 38(10):1095–1102, available from: PM:15461655

Larsen CR, Soerensen JL, Grantcharov TP, Dalsgaard T, Schouenborg L, Ottosen C, Schroeder TV, Ottesen BS (2009) Effect of virtual reality training on laparoscopic surgery: randomised controlled trial. BMJ 338:b1802, available from: PM:19443914

Mabrey JD, Cannon WD, Gillogly SD, Kasser JR, Sweeney HJ, Zarins B, Mevis H, Garrett WE, Poss R (2000) Development of a virtual reality arthroscopic knee simulator. Stud Health Technol Inform 70:192–194, available from: PM:10977538

McCarthy AD, Hollands RJ (1998) A commercially viable virtual reality knee arthroscopy training system. Stud Health Technol Inform 50:302–308, available from: PM:10180558

McCarthy AD, Moody L, Waterworth AR, Bickerstaff DR (2006) Passive haptics in a knee arthroscopy simulator: is it valid for core skills training? Clin Orthop Relat Res 442:13–20, available from: PM:16394733

McGovern KT (1994) Applications of virtual reality to surgery. BMJ 308(6936):1054–1055, available from: PM:8173422

Megali G, Tonet O, Mazzoni M, Dario P, Vascellari A, Marcacci M (2002) A new tool for surgical training in knee arthroscopy. In: Dohi T, Kikinis R (eds), Tokio, pp 170–177. http://link.springer.com/chapter/10.1007%2F3-540-45787-9_22

Megali G, Tonet O, Dario P, Vascellari A, Marcacci M (2005) Computer-assisted training system for knee arthroscopy. Int J Med Robot 1(3):57–66, available from: PM:17518391

Michelson JD (2006) Simulation in orthopaedic education: an overview of theory and practice. J Bone Joint Surg Am 88(6):1405–1411, available from: PM:16757778

Modi CS, Morris G, Mukherjee R (2010) Computer-simulation training for knee and shoulder arthroscopic surgery. Arthroscopy 26(6):832–840, available from: PM:20511043

Moody L, Arthur J, Zivanovic A, Waterworth A (2003) A part-task approach to haptic knee arthroscopy training. Stud Health Technol Inform 94:216–218, available from: PM:15455896

Moody L, Waterworth A, McCarthy AD, Harley P, Smallwood R (2008) The feasibility of a mixed reality surgical training environment. Virtual Reality 12:77–86

Oxford English Dictionary. Oxford University Press. http://www.oed.com. Accessed 15 Jan 2014

Poss R, Mabrey JD, Gillogly SD, Kasser JR, Sweeney HJ, Zarins B, Garrett WE Jr, Cannon WD (2000) Development of a virtual reality arthroscopic knee simulator. J Bone Joint Surg Am 82-A(10):1495–1499, available from: PM:11057478

Riley R (2008) Manual of simulation in healthcare. Oxford University Press, Oxford

Satava RM (1993) Virtual reality surgical simulator. The first steps. Surg Endosc 7(3):203–205, available from: PM:8503081

Satava RM (1994) Emerging medical applications of virtual reality: a surgeon's perspective. Artif Intell Med 6(4):281–288, available from: PM:7812423

Seymour NE, Gallagher AG, Roman SA, O'Brien MK, Bansal VK, Andersen DK, Satava RM (2002) Virtual reality training improves operating room performance: results of a randomized, double-blinded study. Ann Surg 236(4):458–463, available from: PM:12368674

Sherman KP, Ward JW, Wills DP, Mohsen AM (1999) A portable virtual environment knee arthroscopy training system with objective scoring. Stud Health Technol Inform 62:335–336, available from: PM:10538382

Sherman KP, Ward JW, Wills DP, Sherman VJ, Mohsen AM (2001) Surgical trainee assessment using a VE knee arthroscopy training system (VE-KATS): experimental results. Stud Health Technol Inform 81:465–470, available from: PM:11317792

Ward JW, Wills DPM, Sherman KP, Mohsen AMMA (1998) The development of an arthroscopic surgical simulator with haptic feedback. Future Gen Comp Syst 14(3-4):243–251, available from: ISI:000075461200013

Zhou M, Perreault J, Schwaitzberg SD, Cao CG (2008) Effects of experience on force perception threshold in minimally invasive surgery. Surg Endosc 22(2):510–515, available from: PM:17704870

Ziegler R, Fischer G, Muller W, Gobel M (1995) Virtual-reality arthroscopy training simulator. Comput Biol Med 25(2):193–203, available from: ISI:A1995RF80700011

Theory on Simulator Validation

8

Jamie Y. Ferguson, Abtin Alvand, Andrew J. Price, and Jonathan L. Rees

Not everything that counts can be measured, not everything that can be measured counts. – Albert Einstein

Take-Home Messages

- Validation of surgical simulators is a key prerequisite for developing simulation-based surgical education and ensures that teaching and assessment methods are scientifically robust.
- Validation is not a binary concept but involves gathering evidence that a preconceived "construct" holds true in a given context.
- All assessment involves compromise. It is important to understand where these compromises can be made and where they should not.
- The most important aspect of validity is the hardest to measure; that simulation impacts clinical performance and results in improved patient outcomes.

J.Y. Ferguson MB ChB (Hons), MRCS (Ed), MEd (✉)
J.L. Rees, MD
Nuffield Department of Orthopaedics,
Rheumatology and Musculoskeletal Sciences,
University of Oxford, Oxford, UK
e-mail: jamieferguson@doctors.org.uk;
jonathan.rees@ndorms.ox.ac.uk

A. Alvand, BSc(Hons), MBBS, MRCS(Eng)
A.J. Price, MD
Nuffield Department of Orthopaedic Surgery,
Nuffield Orthopaedic Centre, Oxford, UK
e-mail: abtin.alvand@ndorms.ox.ac.uk;
andrew.price@ndorms.ox.ac.uk

8.1 Importance of Developing Simulation-Based Surgical Education

It is argued that traditional apprenticeship training lacks objectivity in the assessment of operative ability (Darzi et al. 1999). The implementation of standardized curricula aims to ensure all trainees achieve critical competencies and so the role of simulation is becoming more important (Motola et al. 2013). It is imperative, however, that any simulation models developed provide a fair reflection of the tasks that they are designed to replicate and their use genuinely improves the relevant skill domains they are aimed at improving.

In this chapter, we will introduce some of the important concepts in ensuring simulation is valid and useful. We will look at some of the theory underpinning how new simulation technologies can be evaluated to ensure they deliver in their intended applications specifically within arthroscopic training.

Given the high costs associated with introducing simulation-based technologies into training curricula, the process of validation is an important one as it attempts to establish whether or not the intended simulators are able to deliver on some of their claims. Several concepts need to be understood including validity and reliability.

M. Karahan et al. (eds.), *Effective Training of Arthroscopic Skills*,
DOI 10.1007/978-3-662-44943-1_8, © ESSKA 2015

8.2   Validity

Validity is a fundamental property of a test or assessment tool and is concerned with whether or not it measures what it purports to measure (Gallagher et al. 2003). Validity is not a characteristic of the simulation model itself but of the theoretical framework (otherwise known as the "construct") used in the model's application (Aucar et al. 2005). In other words, validity is related to the way in which the simulation model is used, rather than being an inherent property of the simulator itself. Simulation-based training models could be used in many different ways. Examples include an aid to training, a way of assessing progress or as a high-stakes competency assessment. In all of these applications, the simulation tool may remain the same, but the construct is different because the way that the simulation is applied and interpreted varies (Clauser et al. 2008; Scalese and Hatala 2013).

It is a common misconception that once validity is proven for a simulation model, it acts as a blanket term, applying to all other possible applications of that simulator. Instead each particular application of the simulation model has a specific construct that relates to that particular application. Any changing in the way the simulation model is used will result in a change in the construct and as a result may not be supported by the previous validation process. When designing a simulation tool, it is important that a clear decision is made regarding its intended role or purpose. If a simulation tool is used within a different context or in a different way to that which it was first conceived, its validity must again be demonstrated with further testing (Sedlack 2011). Validity should not be thought of as a binary concept but as a spectrum. Rather than being merely present or absent, there are degrees of validity, determined by the weight of supporting evidence available for that test. Proving perfect validity for any test is probably unachievable in the real world. Validation studies aim to provide sufficient evidence to support the construct as providing a true measure of what is tested within a specific context.

Any confusion surrounding the concept of validity may be related to the many different definitions discussed in the literature. Despite the various terms described for validity, it is in fact a singular entity. The various types described refer to slightly different facets of the same single concept (Garden 2008).

In the classical model of validity, three principle components of validity were described, namely, content validity, criterion-orientated validity, and construct validity (Cronbach and Meehl 1955). Various other facets of validity are grouped under these three principle headings (as outlined in Table 8.1) (Carter et al. 2005; Garden 2008; Michelson 2006).

Table 8.1 Forms of validity

(1) *Content validity*	
Evidence that the items of the simulation reflect the domain being tested. Each content area that is related to the construct should be included	
(a) Face	Subjective impression by non-experts of how closely the simulation replicates the real environment
(b) Content	Ensuring the simulation covers all the important components of a task as determined by expert opinion
(2) *Criterion-orientated validity*	
The relationship of performance in the new simulation compared to other independent established measures of the ability in the domain of interest	
(a) Concurrent	Correlation with an independent measure of ability performed at the same time as the simulation
(b) Predictive	Ability of the simulation to predict future performance by correlation with future test score
(3) *Construct validity*	
The overarching concept supported by all other forms of validity. It is the degree to which the simulation measures the theoretical construct. In other words, does the simulation measure arthroscopic ability, or does it merely measure the ability to perform the simulated task	
(a) Discriminant	The ability of the simulation to discriminate between those with differing abilities (such as junior and senior trainees)
(b) Convergent	The ability of the simulation to not differentiate between individuals of similar ability

More recently, there has been growing dissatisfaction with these categories which some feel make arbitrary distinctions between different forms of validity that do not really exist. The more modern view of validity is that it is a unitary concept without differing forms. Contemporary authors have proposed that in psychometric testing, these three distinct themes should be subsumed into the more comprehensive overarching theme of *construct validity* (American Educational Research Association et al. 1999).

8.3   Face Validity

Face validity is increasingly sidelined within validation processes. It is a subjective measure of how closely a simulation resembles real life and is usually measured through questioning experts. This is often a basic prerequisite of designing simulation-based studies or tasks, and is not really a part of validity testing. As Downing and Haladyna note, "*the appearance of validity is not validity*," (Downing and Haladyna 2004). However, a high degree of face validity can positively influence the *acceptance* of simulation-based tasks by end users – especially among trainee surgeons.

8.4   Content Validity

This looks at the components of a test or simulation and ensures that all the appropriate areas are covered effectively and are relevant to the test. It ensures the steps within the task are thought out and linked. Often during a simulation's design phase, this process is performed using cognitive task analysis when an expert is asked to talk through a task so that the various steps can be noted down by the developers with the ultimate aim of their incorporation into the simulation scenario. This form of validity is also relatively subjective, often relying on expert opinion.

8.5   Construct Validity

This is the ability of a test to identify and measure the attributes of performance it is designed to measure such that it is able to differentiate between novices and experts. There can be no argument that a simulation task for knee arthroscopy that cannot distinguish between expert surgeons and junior trainees possesses little validity as an assessment tool. Furthermore, construct validity must be reassessed as new/further skill metrics are discovered, in order to ensure the model is a fair representation of what is being tested.

8.6   Concurrent Validity

This is achieved by using other measurements of ability and correlating them with the simulation. This process is often employed when introducing a new assessment tool so that it can be compared to the current gold standard assessment. An example might be linking motion analysis movement data (e.g., hand path length) with global rating scales (Alvand et al. 2013). High correlation between different assessment tools indicates good concurrent validity. This process of using multiple data to establish validity is often termed triangulation.

8.7   Discriminate Validity

This involves ensuring that there is no correlation between aspects of the test that should not correlate. In other words it confirms that unrelated parts of a test are in actual fact unrelated. In the context of simulation, it means that the parameters are able to differentiate between established experts and novices.

8.8   Convergent Validity

This is the counterpart to discriminate validity. This is the ability of a test to demonstrate that elements that should be related are related.

An example in simulation is the ability of a test to show that individuals of a similar skill level are grouped together appropriately.

8.9   Predictive Validity

This is the ability of a simulation/simulated task/simulator to predict actual performance in the real clinical setting from the simulated performance. This is probably the most important aspect of validity testing, but in reality little literature has looked at this in arthroscopic simulation and it is one of the most challenging aspects to prove (Hodgins and Veillette 2013; Slade Shantz et al. 2014). Long-term transferability studies are necessary for predictive validity to be established. Furthermore, a reliable way of assessing operative ability is required so as to compare performance in real-life settings with simulation performance. In addition, it is important to remember that technical ability is only one of a number of influences on patient outcome. Spencer stated that surgery is 75 % decision-making and 25 % dexterity (Spencer 1978). Daley and coworkers identified several other factors that contribute to the quality of surgical care including, leadership, which technology is used, the interface with other services and institutions, the level of the coordination of work, and how quality of care is monitored (Daley et al. 1997). Therefore, although it is highly desirable to link technical skill scores and clinical outcome, the large number of *nontechnical* factors that influence patient outcome make identifying a correlation very challenging.

8.10   Sources of validity evidence

As previously stated, validity is a unitary concept and the various aspects of validity discussed are not distinct types but different forms of evidence accumulated to support the intended interpretation of performance for the proposed purpose (American Educational Research Association, American Psychological Association, and National Council on Measurement in Education 1999). Evidence for a construct's validity

can be gathered in five different domains outlined in Table 8.2 (American Educational Research Association, American Psychological

Table 8.2 The five elements of construct validity as outlined by Messick (Messick 1989; Messick 1995)

Types of evidence for validity (Messick 1989)	Description
Content	This is a measure of the extent to which a test's content assesses the skill domain that it purports to assess/measure. This involves ensuring that all the relevant aspects of the task assessed are included to avoid the problem of "underrepresentation" as well as avoiding the risk of "construct-irrelevance" (a situation where factors irrelevant to the construct are measured). This is usually achieved through expert opinion on the test contents
Response process	This ensures the fit between the construct and the performance of the test. For example, scores in a mathematical test of higher-order thinking should be different between those who actually use higher-order thinking and those who have simply memorized the answers. Ensuring this may involve asking test takers to "show their working" or demonstrate their thought process. It also encapsulates rater scoring, ensuring judgments are not made based on irrelevant factors, such as how the candidate is dressed
Internal structure	Scores that are intended to measure a single construct should deliver homogenous results where individuals with varying ability should attain scores that can allow discrimination between them. This is also used as a test to ensure reliability by testing internal consistency
Relation to other variables	Correlation with other instruments where observed relationships match with predicted relationships or a lack of correlation where it is not expected would support this. The instruments used, such as motion analysis or global rating scales, would also need to have been previously validated for use in this way

Table 8.2 (continued)

Types of evidence for validity (Messick 1989)	Description
Consequences of testing	These are the intended and unintended consequences of testing. For example, trainees may only concentrate on elements of the curriculum that are tested while neglecting other topics. Another example might be using a simulator for selection from an unrelated domain. If a flight simulator was used for selection into higher surgical training, this process may have questionable validity

Association, and National Council on Measurement in Education 1999; Cook and Beckman 2006; Downing 2003; Messick 1989).

8.11   Threats to Validity

There are two principle threats to validity that must be avoided, namely,

> *construct underrepresentation* and *construct-irrelevant variance*. (Messick 1995).

Construct underrepresentation refers to the degree to which the assessment fails to capture important aspects of the construct. This will have an impact on the score interpretations, as the evidence they are based on will be weak if important aspects of the construct are not tested. An example of this might be trying to use an isolated plastic synthetic bone model without soft tissue cover to test competence at performing open reduction internal fixation of a tibial plateau fracture. Although this model would be good at assessing procedural knowledge, not simulating the soft tissues overlying the bone would greatly reduce the validity of the task as the sole test of competence for this complex procedure.

Construct-irrelevant variance refers to the degree to which extraneous or irrelevant factors impact upon the test score. This may be systematic, such as from bias, or a result of the testing scenario being so broad that it incorporates elements irrelevant to the tested construct.

This generates "noise" making the interpretation of the results more difficult. Poor design of the simulation instrument can make this problem worse if the performance of some users is improved by extraneous clues or prompts in the test format that are irrelevant to the construct or if some are disadvantaged for reasons outside the construct of interest.

8.12   Reliability

Reliability refers to the consistency or stability of measurement in a test (Kazdin 2003). It is the measure of the reproducibility of test scores obtained from an assessment given multiple times under the same conditions. All measurement has inherent variability, and the difference between a single measurement and the "true" measurement is termed the measurement error (Boulet and Murray 2012). All assessment involves taking a sample of an individual's knowledge or performance and making inferences about that data to reach a conclusion about the individual's true ability. The greater the difference between the assessment result and the individual's true ability, the less reliable the assessment. A reliable test gives a fair reflection of an individual's true ability.

The concepts of reliability and validity are intrinsically linked, and their relationship can be illustrated using the analogy of hitting archery targets (Fig. 8.1). Reliability is a necessary, but not sufficient component of validity (Cook and Beckman 2006). If the components of a test are unreliable, then conclusions cannot be drawn from the results, and the test is no longer valid. For example, if a new simulator is used to assess an experienced surgeon's operative ability and of four repetitions it rates his performance as "average," "very poor," "excellent," and "good," the test can be seen to lack reliability. Conversely, if the simulation result was consistently "poor," then although the test could be called reliable (due to the consistent results over multiple tests) it would lack validity, assuming that there was sufficient objective evidence that the surgeon really possessed expert surgical skills. Only when the test consistently rates his performance as excellent could the simulator be said to be both reliable and valid.

a   b

c   d

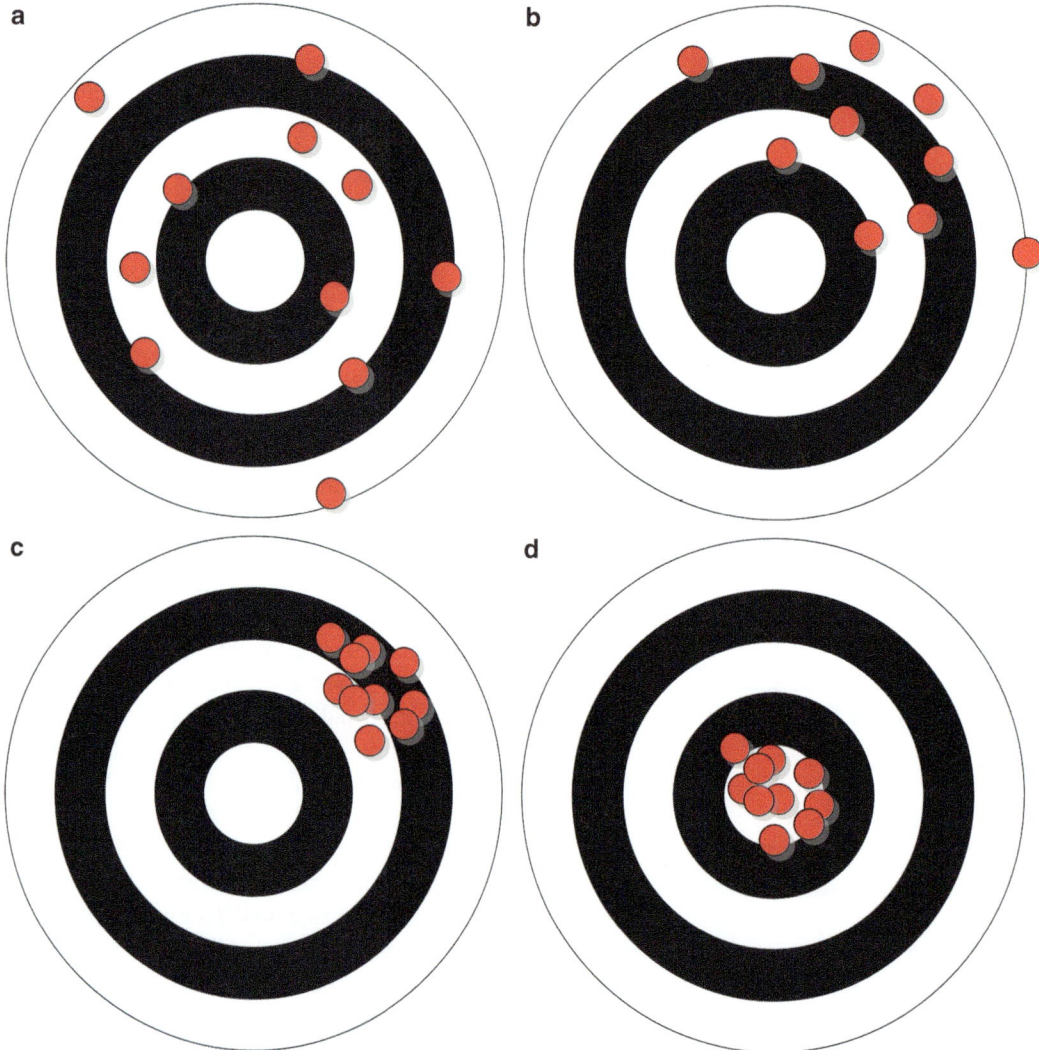

Fig. 8.1 Validity and reliability are intrinsically linked. Imagine each shot represents a test score and the bull's eye represents a candidate's true ability. (**a**) Shots centred around bull's eye but spread out, therefore valid but not reliable. (**b**) Shots not centred around Bull's eye and spread out, therefore not valid or reliable. (**c**) Reliable but not valid. (**d**) Valid and reliable

Assuming the measurement error is equally distributed, the reliability of an assessment should be improved by increasing the sampling (Downing 2004). This is because with sufficient repetition of assessment, the error should average towards zero. This can be achieved by making the test longer, increasing the number of different assessment parameters or by increasing the number of raters. The degree of measurement error impacts on how long a test must be to achieve adequate reliability and will therefore determine the values of any single measurement (Garden 2008).

In psychometric testing, it is often not practical to obtain multiple measurements of an individual to correct for high measurement errors. Therefore designing simulators with good reliability is important, particularly if they are to be used for assessment. This is especially true for high-stakes assessment (such as for licensing and certification assessment which are designed to protect real patients from incompetence) where the consequences of a false positive result may cause patient harm. Reliability can be measured in several ways as outlined in Table 8.3.

Table 8.3 The various aspects of reliability testing

Type of reliability evidence	Description
Test-retest	Otherwise known as intrasubject reliability, this measures if trainees achieve similar scores on two different occasions
Internal consistency	This is assessed by comparing the relationship between different elements of the test or simulation. Correlations can be measured between each item of the test, known as inter-item correlation, or by dividing the test into two parts and comparing them, known as split-half correlation. Poor correlation may suggest that more than one construct is being measured
Parallel forms	If the test items for the content of interest are randomly divided into two separate tests and administered to subjects at the same time, there should be strong correlation
Inter-rater	This test ensures that there is good agreement between assessors of a trainee's performance. Two forms exist: interobserver reliability measures the agreement between different assessors for a given test, whereas intraobserver reliability determines the variability of a single assessor's marks for the same test on different occasions

8.13   Statistically Measuring Reliability

8.13.1 Cronbach Alpha

The most common method of determining the reliability of an assessment tool is by use of the Cronbach Alpha (Cronbach 1951). This is a test of internal consistency, and it calculates the correlation between all the test items in all possible combinations. It can be expressed as

$$\alpha = \frac{n}{n-1}\left(1 - \frac{\Sigma Vi}{V_{test}}\right)$$

where n is the number of test elements, Vi is a measure of the variance of the score on each test element, and V_{test} is the total variance of all scores on the whole assessment.

A shortcut for estabilising the degree of variance for each test item can be calculated using the following formula:

$$Vi = Pi \times (1 - Pi)$$

where Pi is the percentage of candidates who correctly perform the test element (expressed as a decimal). This will always give a number between 0-0.25.

Cronbach alpha generates a score between 0 and 1 to give a coefficient of internal consistency. The figure required will depend on the context of the assessment. For high-stakes tests, such as licensing exams, a figure of 0.9 or above is preferred, but for other forms of assessment, values of 0.7–0.8 may be acceptable (Downing 2004).

One of the strongest methods of improving reliability of a test is to lengthen the assessment by including more test items. This can be seen from the formula where the biggest impact on reliability is the V_{test} item because the larger the value, the higher the α score. For example, if we were to double the length of the assessment, the V_{test} will increase by a power of four because variance involves a squared term. In contrast the ΣVi will only double because each Vi is just a number between 0 and 0.25. As V_{test} increases faster than ΣVi, the alpha score will increase by virtue of lengthening the test. Therefore, it is important that any simulated task is of sufficient length to ensure reliability.

8.13.2   Standard Error of Measurement (SEM)

This is another less commonly used measure of reliability. It scores the degree of variance in candidate scores by the following formula (Harvill 1991):

$$SEM = \text{Standard Deviation} \times \sqrt{(1 - \text{reliability})}$$

It represents the standard deviation of an individual's scores (American Educational Research Association, American Psychological Association, and National Council on Measurement in Education 1999) and gives an indication of the degree of certainty of the true score from the observed score. A confidence interval can be generated for the candidate's true score such that 95 % of an individual's retest scores should fall within 2 SEM of the true score (Harvill 1991).

8.13.3 Intrasubject Reliability

When using test-retest methods, the correlation between results is usually arrived upon using Pearson's R correlation test. This is generally a more conservative estimate of reliability than Cronbach alpha. However, the practicalities of using this technique are more challenging as it requires two separate sittings of the assessment. Other confounding factors resulting from changes in the conditions of the two assessments must be anticipated and controlled for, such as the potential learning effect from taking the initial test.

8.13.4 Inter-rater Reliability

Obtaining multiple scores is an important component of reliability. All too often scoring of performance is made based on single assessments or by single raters. It has been stated that "a person with one watch knows what time it is, a person with two watches is never quite sure" (Brennan 2010). This illustrates the potential difficulty of using multiple raters. However, increasing the number of assessors is one way on increasing reliability. The correlation between different raters can be measured in several different ways. The simplest is by assessing the percentage agreement between raters. The criticism of this method is that it does not take into account the possibility of agreement through chance alone. Cohen's kappa coefficient is a method for measuring agreement between two observers using a categorical assessment scale (Cohen 1960). It generates a value between -1 and 1 (although negative values are rarely generated and are of little significance in assessment validation). A value of 0 denotes no agreement, and 1 denotes perfect agreement. Figures above 0.6 suggest moderate agreement and above 0.8 suggest strong agreement (McHugh

2012). When comparing performance using an ordinal scale such as a Likert scale, a variation called the weighted kappa is used, which penalizes wider differences in scores between raters than narrower disagreements (Cohen 1968). If more than two raters are used, Fleiss' kappa should be employed (Fleiss 1971). The nonparametric Kendall tau test can be used if assessors use an assessment that involves ranking candidates or data (Cook and Beckman 2006; Sullivan 2011).

8.13.5 Generalizability Theory (G-Theory)

This is another more modern method of estimating reliability using factorial analysis of variance (Brennan 2010; Cook and Beckman 2006). It is able to look at the many sources of error within testing (termed facets) that influence the reliability of performance assessments. The impact of these various facets (such as item variance, rater variance, or subject variance) can be quantified, and the source and magnitude of the variability can be measured (Cook and Beckman 2006). This allows researchers to ask what factors have the greatest impact on reliability as well as helping to determine how to improve reliability though altering various error effects. For example, it may show that the greatest impact on reliability is the variation in inter-rater scoring. In this situation, this would tell us that the generalizability of the test across more observers is likely to be reduced.

8.14 Simulation Utility Involves Compromise

Van de Vleuten proposed that rather than thinking of factors such as reliability and validity in isolation, the most important overall measure of an instrument is its "utility" (Van der Vleuten 1996). This is a product of several different elements that all contribute to how useful it is in practice. As well as reliability and validity, these factors include educational impact, acceptability, and cost. In the real world, it is impossible to produce the perfect simulation due to the limitation of resources such as time and cost. Consequently, all constructs require compromise to be feasible. Understanding this reality allows careful consideration of where the greatest compromise can be made which will depend upon what the main purpose of the simulation is envisaged to be. If the simulation is designed for a high-stakes assessment of competency, then reliability cannot be compromised to ensure no unsafe trainee is allowed to progress incorrectly. However, if the simulation is designated as a training tool that gives feedback for learning, reliability is less important, with efforts made to limit compromising validity, so that feedback is ensured to be of relevance to the task in question.

Test utility is therefore a function of all these factors and can be expressed in the conceptual model as follows (Van der Vleuten 1996):

$$Utility = Reliability \times Validity \times Educational\,impact \times Acceptability \times Cost$$

8.15 How to Practically Ensure Validity

Kane proposed a framework for evaluating the validity of a construct. This involves a chain of inferences to develop a validity argument (Kane 1992; Kane 2001; Kane 2006).

First, the proposed interpretive argument for a construct should be stated as clearly and explicitly as possible. Next, all available evidence for and against the validity argument can be investigated, and a coherent argument for the proposed interpretation of scores can be developed, as well as arguments against plausible alternate explanations. As a result of these evaluations, the interpretive argument may be rejected, or it may be improved by adapting the interpretation or measurement techniques to correct any problems identified. If the interpretive argument survives all reasonable challenges, it can be accepted provisionally, with the caveat that further factors may come to light in the future that challenge this argument.

This chain of inferences has four principle links that extend from simulation implementation to result interpretation. These are *scoring*, *generalization*, *extrapolation*, and *decision*.

8.15.1 Scoring

This concerns how observations on a participant's performance are made and how this performance is converted into a score. It evaluates if the simulation is reproducibly administered under standard conditions and includes scrutinizing the scoring rubrics, ensuring that they are applied constantly to all candidates and safeguarding security of the assessment so that no candidates gain an unfair advantage. One of the strengths of simulation assessment is that it can provide a standardized testing environment to all candidates. However, potential threats to this first inference can occur, including such things as simulation malfunction or vague scoring criteria. Validity evidence that addresses these issues might include regular checks and calibration of simulators and appropriate design and scrutiny of marking sheets by experts to ensure marking is homogenous.

8.15.2 Generalization

This concerns the inference that the performance tested is representative of the "universe" of scores that could be obtained in similar tasks. In other words, are the scores sufficiently representative of all other possible observations? The main threat to this is construct underrepresentation. Most simulations contain a relatively small number of items, which means making inferences about performance in the real world from simulation can be risky. Ensuring the simulation is constructed suitably and that appropriate sampling of the construct is undertaken will limit this issue. This inference also encompasses issues of reliability, internal consistency, and sources of measurement error. One of the ways of strengthening the generalization inference is to increase the number of items tested. One of the strengths of simulation is that additional targeted models can be developed to ensure the breadth of surgical performance is covered. This could be achieved by generating simulation lists, when trainees can perform several different simulations is one sitting, much like a regular operating list.

8.15.3 Extrapolation

This inference is principally concerned with the extrapolation of simulation performance to real-world performance. This can be gauged by looking at the correlation between simulation scores and measures of real-life clinical performance. For example, there is a more robust argument that a knee arthroscopy simulation is able to predict real-life ability if experienced knee surgeons performed better than trainees. This represents construct validity (by demonstrating an ability to differentiate between surgeons of differing experience levels), and it is a key component of the extrapolation inference. Through a process termed "triangulation," other direct or indirect markers of ability can also be used in combination to strengthen this inference. Such an example is the use of motion tracking systems. Other measures that could be selected might include the results of in-training exams, OSCE scores, seniority, or other similar studies (Sullivan 2011).

8.15.4 Decision Making

When judgments are made about technical ability from simulation performance, cut scores are required to determine if individuals meet the required standard. It is important that the setting of these standards of pass and fail are robust and defensible (Boulet et al. 2003). Moreover, the wishes of other stakeholders impacted by these decisions must also be considered. Even if strong evidence exists of a simulator's validity from the three other inferences outlined already, if those to whom the results are important do not believe them to be credible or meaningful, then they are not valid (Scalese and Hatala 2013). For example, the general public would probably dismiss the credibility of a simulation assessment that allowed poorly performing surgeons to pass through without being identified and call its validity into question.

8.16 Discussion

Simulation training is an exciting area, with much potential for use in training orthopedic surgeons of the future. However, for its potential to be realized, it must be feasible, and its implementation must ensure simulated tasks and assessment systems have adequate reliability and validity.

In this chapter, we have discussed the various elements of validity desirable in simulation. Validity is a broad concept with many facets and should involve the accumulation of a variety of evidence to construct a strong validation argument. Careful thought is needed prior to this process to identify the simulation's application. It is important that future developers aim to coordinate their efforts with policy makers, those writing the curricula and simulation model manufacturers so that alignment is achieved between simulation and critical learning objectives. This would ensure that future training programs have a common theme and simulation is delivered with clear aims and in an effective manner (Table 8.4).

Table 8.4 Checklist for simulation validation

Checklist for validating simulation
1. Determine the construct
State the aims of the simulator. The construct's form will depend of several factors, such as:
(a) *What will its purpose be?*
e.g. introducing junior trainees to arthroscopy or high-stakes certification exams at the end of training
(b) *How will it be applied?*
(c) *Under what conditions will the simulation take place?*
(d) *What will it measure? What are the outcome parameters?*
Performance metrics e.g. time taken, motion analysis
Rater scoring e.g. checklists, rating scales or subjective assessment
End product
(e) *What group of people will it be used with?*
If various groups are to use the simulator, validation must include these groups
(f) *What type of model will be used?*
Phantom model/benchtop model
Cadaveric
Virtual reality
Simulated patient actors
(g) *What evidence is there within the literature for this simulation modality?*
2. Content evidence
(a) Expert panel
Was there expert consensus on the construct design including formal task analysis?
(b) Instrument validation
Are new instruments based on previously validated instruments?
(c) Pilot testing
Have the simulation instruments been developed and revised through piloting and modified as appropriate?
(d) Score framework
What evidence was used to determine scoring methods and can a scoring blueprint be prepared?
(e) Test blueprinting
Is a blueprint used to develop test instruments?
(f) Evidence of content-construct mismatch
Is there any discrepancy between alignment of test content and the construct?
3. Reliability tests
(a) Test/retest
(b) Internal consistency
(c) Inter-/intra-rater reliability
4. Test consequences
(a) *How will test thresholds be established?*
e.g. Angoff method, modified borderline group method, Markov modeling, ROC curve
(b) *Have unanticipated test consequences been considered?*
5. Feasibility
(a) Ethical considerations and institutional approval
(b) Consideration of cost implication for local unit
6. Educational issues
Establish how learner feedback is to be delivered:
Metrics such as time taken, instrument path length, etc.
Video
Performance score e.g. check list, scoring rubric, GRS, etc.
One-to-one debriefing with experienced surgeon
7. Predictive validity
Establish correlation of performance in real-world environment with simulation performance

Bibliography

Alvand A, Logishetty K, Middleton R, Khan T, Jackson WF, Price AJ, Rees JL (2013) Validating a global rating scale to monitor individual resident learning curves during arthroscopic knee meniscal repair. Arthroscopy 29(5):906–912

American Educational Research Association, American Psychological Association, National Council on Measurement in Education (1999) Standards for educational and psychological testing. American Educational Research Association, Washington

Aucar JA, Groch NR, Troxel SA, Eubanks SW (2005) A review of surgical simulation with attention to validation methodology. Surg Laparosc Endosc Percutan Tech 15(2):82–89

Boulet JR, De Champlain AF, McKinley DW (2003) Setting defensible performance standards on osces and standardized patient examinations. Med Teach 25(3): 245–249

Brennan RL (2010) Generalizability theory. Springer, New York

Carter FJ, Schijven MP, Aggarwal R, Grantcharov T, Francis NK, Hanna GB, Jakimowicz JJ (2005) Consensus guidelines for validation of virtual reality surgical simulators. Surg Endosc 19(12):1523–1532

Chikwe J, De Souza AC, Pepper JR (2004) No time to train the surgeons. Br Med J 328(7437):418–419

Clauser BE, Margolis MJ, Swanson DB (2008) Issues of validity and reliability for assessments in medical education. In: Practical guide to the evaluation of clinical competence. p 10–23

Cohen J (1960) A coefficient of agreement for nominal scales. Educ Psychol Meas 20(1):37–46

Cohen J (1968) Weighted kappa: Nominal scale agreement provision for scaled disagreement or partial credit. Psychol Bull 70(4):213–220

Cook DA, Beckman TJ (2006) Current concepts in validity and reliability for psychometric instruments: theory and application. Am J Med 119(2):166.e7–116.e16

Cronbach LJ (1951) Coefficient alpha and the internal structure of tests. Psychometrika 16(3):297–334

Cronbach LJ, Meehl PE (1955) Construct validity in psychological tests. Psychol Bull 52(4):281–302

Daley J, Forbes MG, Young GJ, Charns MP, Gibbs JO, Hur K et al (1997) Validating risk-adjusted surgical outcomes: site visit assessment of process and structure. J Am Coll Surg 185(4):341–351

Darzi A, Smith S, Taffinder N (1999) Assessing operative skill: needs to become more objective. Br Med J 318(7188):887–888

Downing SM (2003) Validity: on the meaningful interpretation of assessment data. Med Educ 37(9):830–837

Downing SM (2004) Reliability: on the reproducibility of assessment data. Med Educ 38(9):1006–1012

Downing SM, Haladyna TM (2004) Validity threats: overcoming interference with proposed interpretations of assessment data. Med Educ 38(3):327–333

Fleiss JL (1971) Measuring nominal scale agreement among many raters. Psychol Bull 76(5):378–382

Gallagher AG, Ritter EM, Satava RM (2003) Fundamental principles of validation, and reliability: rigorous science for the assessment of surgical education and training. Surg Endosc 17(10):1525–1529

Garden A (2008) Research in simulation. In: Riley RH (ed) Manual of simulation in healthcare. Oxford University Press, New York

Harvill LM (1991) Standard error of measurement. Educ Measure Issues Pract 10(2):33–41

Hodges B, Regehr G, McNaughton N, Tiberius R, Hanson M (1999) OSCE checklists do not capture increasing levels of expertise. Acad Med 74(10):1129–1134

Hodges B, McNaughton N, Regehr G, Tiberius R, Hanson M (2002) The challenge of creating new OSCE measures to capture the characteristics of expertise. Med Educ 36(8):742–748

Hodgins JL, Veillette C (2013) Arthroscopic proficiency: methods in evaluating competency. BMC Med Educ 13(1):61–69

Holmboe ES, Sherbino J, Long DM, Swing SR, Frank JR (2010) The role of assessment in competency-based medical education. Med Teach 32(8):676–682

Jarvis-Selinger S, Pratt DD, Regehr G (2012) Competency is not enough: integrating identity formation into the medical education discourse. Acad Med 87(9):1185–1190

Kane MT (1992) The assessment of professional competence. Eval Health Prof 15(2):163–182

Kane MT (2001) Current concerns in validity theory. J Educ Measure 38(4):319–342

Kane M (2006) Validation. In: Brennan RL (ed) Educational measurement. ACE/Praeger, Westport, pp 7–64

Kassab E, Tun JK, Kneebone RL (2012) A novel approach to contextualized surgical simulation training. Simul Healthc 7(3):155–161

Kazdin AE (2003) Research design in clinical psychology, 4th edn. Pearson

Kneebone R (2009) Perspective: simulation and transformational change: the paradox of expertise. Acad Med 84(7):954–957

Kunkler K (2006) The role of medical simulation: an overview. Int J Med Robot 2(3):203–210

Martin JA, Regehr G, Reznick R, MacRae H, Murnaghan J, Hutchison C, Brown M (1997) Objective structured assessment of technical skill (OSATS) for surgical residents. Br J Surg 84(2):273–278

McHugh ML (2012) Interrater reliability: the kappa statistic. Biochem Med 22(3):276–282

Mehay R, Burns R (2009) Available from: http://www.bradfordvts.co.uk/wp-content/onlineresources/0002mrcgp/mrcgp%20in%20a%20nutshell.ppt. Accessed 20 Jan 2014

Messick S (1989) Validity. In: Linn RL (ed) Educational measurement. American Council on Education/Macmillan, New York, pp 13–103

Messick S (1995) Validity of psychological assessment: validation of inferences from persons' responses and performances as scientific inquiry into score meaning. Am Psychol 50(9):741–749

Michelson JD (2006) Simulation in orthopaedic education: an overview of theory and practice. J Bone Joint Surg 88(6):1405–1411

Miller GE (1990) The assessment of clinical skills/competence/performance. Acad Med 65(9):S63–S67

Motola I, Devine LA, Chung HS, Sullivan JE, Issenberg SB (2013) Simulation in healthcare education: a best evidence practical guide. AMEE guide no. 82. Med Teach 35(10):e1511–e1530

Murray D (2012) Review article: assessment in anesthesiology education. Can J Anesth 59(2):182–192

Regehr G, MacRae H, Reznick RK, Szalay D (1998) Comparing the psychometric properties of checklists and global rating scales for assessing performance on an osce-format examination. Acad Med 73(9):993–997

Sadideen H, Hamaoui K, Saadeddin M, Kneebone R (2012) Simulators and the simulation environment: getting the balance right in simulation-based surgical education. Int J Surg 10:458–462

Scalese RJ, Hatala R (2013) Competency assessment. In: Levine AI, DeMaria S, Schwartz AD, Sim AJ (eds)

The comprehensive textbook of healthcare simulation. Springer, New York

Schuwirth LW, Van Der Vleuten CP (2004) Changing education, changing assessment, changing research? Med Educ 38(8):805–812

Sedlack RE (2011) Validation process for new endoscopy teaching tools. Tech Gastrointest Endosc 13(2):151–154

Shantz JAS, Leiter JR, Gottschalk T, MacDonald PB (2014) The internal validity of arthroscopic simulators and their effectiveness in arthroscopic education. Knee Surg Sports Traumatol Arthrosc 22:33–40

Spencer F (1978) Teaching and measuring surgical techniques: the technical evaluation of competence. Bull Am Coll Surg 63(3):9–12

Sullivan GM (2011) A primer on the validity of assessment instruments. J Grad Med Educ 3(2):119–120

Van Der Vleuten CP (1996) The assessment of professional competence: developments, research and practical implications. Adv Health Sci Educ 1(1):41–67

Wass V, Vleuten CVD, Shatzer J, Jones R (2001) Assessment of clinical competence. Lancet 357(9260):945–949

Simulator Evaluation

9

Gabriëlle J.M. Tuijthof and Jonathan L. Rees

Take-Home Messages

- Simulator evaluation is dependent on the wishes of the community (Chap. 2), the general requirements for medical simulators and validation (Chap. 8).
- Simulator validation is a precondition that ensures useful and appropriate skills training.
- Higher-quality studies are still required to show the validity of most simulators.
- Standardisation of validation protocols and training tasks would allow objective comparison between different simulators.
- At present, the most validated simulators are Procedicus™ virtual reality shoulder joint and the Sawbones™ anatomic knee bench model.

G.J.M. Tuijthof (✉)
Department of Biomechanical Engineering,
Delft University of Technology, Delft,
The Netherlands

Department of Orthopedic Surgery,
Academic Medical Centre, Amsterdam,
The Netherlands
e-mail: g.j.m.tuijthof@tudelft.nl

J.L. Rees, MD
Nuffield Department of Orthopaedics, Rheumatology
and Musculoskeletal Sciences, University of Oxford,
Oxford, UK
e-mail: jonathan.rees@ndorms.ox.ac.uk

9.1 Requirements for Simulator Evaluation

Validation is a very important, but not the sole criterion based upon which simulators should be evaluated. In this chapter, we propose three sets of evaluation criteria to assess the appropriateness of simulators to train arthroscopic skills: wishes from the arthroscopic community (Chap. 2), general requirements for medical simulators and validation (Chap. 8). The first two sets of criteria are elucidated in the remainder of this section; the latter is fully covered in Chap. 8. *For the simulators presented in* Chaps. 5, 6, and 7, we evaluate to what extent they fulfil these three sets of criteria. This will be done using a 3-point Likert scale: + implies the simulator completely fulfils a requirement, ~ implies that the simulator fulfils a requirement to some extent and – implies that the simulator does not fulfil a requirement. Whenever possible, the evaluation is performed per type of simulator, for example, high-fidelity virtual reality simulators or box trainers (see classification Chap. 6).

9.2 Wishes from the Arthroscopy Community

In Chap. 2, an inventory held amongst the ESSKA members is presented indicating the necessary tasks and skills that should be trained in a simulated environment away from the patient, before training in the operating room continues. As was shown, some of the skills do not require actual instrument handling (e.g. knowledge on anatomy) or a simulator per se (e.g. patient positioning). These skills are omitted in this chapter, which solely focuses on the arthroscopic skills training that do require a simulator. Therefore, we propose to evaluate the different types of simulators on their appropriateness to enable training of the following top five specific skills:

1. Precise portal placement
2. Triangulating the tip of the probe with a 30° scope
3. Insertion of the arthroscope
4. Entry of all compartments (medial/lateral/posteromedial, suprapatellar/intercondylar)
5. Identification of all relevant structures in the knee joint (medial compartment, intercondylar notch, lateral compartment, lateral gutter, medial gutter)

9.3 General Requirements for Medical Simulators

The potential of arthroscopic simulators to be or become a valuable training modality also depends on them fulfilling the general requirements for medical simulators. These requirements are based on an extensive literature review by Issenberg and co-workers (Issenberg et al. 2005) that was updated by McGaghie and co-workers (McGaghie et al. 2010). This list of ten items is presented in order of importance:

Providing feedback
Repetitive practice
Curriculum integration[1]
Range of difficulty level
Multiple learning strategies (see additional information Chaps. 3 and 4)

Capture clinical variation
Controlled environment
Individualised learning
Defined outcomes
Simulator validity[2]

9.4 Evaluation of Wishes and General Requirements

Analysis of Table 9.1 indicates that none of the available simulators offers the capability to train the top five of required arthroscopic skills that a resident should possess before continuing their training in the operating room. Only the anatomic bench models with replaceable skins allow training of precise portal placing. Care has to be taken that each trainee needs to palpate the knee before creating their own set of portals. Of course, when training on cadaver knee joints, the first trainee that starts also has the opportunity to create a set of portals, but those following do not. As box trainers do not represent a realistic knee joint environment, they only train triangulation skills. This is the main arthroscopic skill that can be practiced on all simulators. Triangulation is a core arthroscopic skill, and it is important to practice, since the required eye–hand coordination is different from eye–hand coordination used in daily life. Additionally, all training systems that offer a human joint environment to train in allow training of the entry to compartments and identification of anatomic structures (Table 9.1). A challenge of virtual reality simulators is offering the realistic haptic feedback, especially in tasks such as the insertion of arthroscope. To increase realism of haptic sensation, high-fidelity virtual simulators now have a passive physical model of the joint (McCarthy et al. 2006; Moody et al. 2008).

As cadavers differ per sample, they do not offer a truly controlled environment where repetition of exercises can be practiced over and over (Table 9.2).

[1] We have interpreted this requirement as the simulator offering a high usability that is being 'user friendly', which implies that no manual is required to handle the simulator, and 'easy to use', which implies that no preparation time is required to start training.

[2] As indicated, simulator validation will be discussed in a separate section, where the literature has been reported most extensively on this requirement.

Table 9.1 Crosstab within the left column the top five arthroscopic skills that need to be trained prior to start training in the operating room and in the top row different types of training systems

Skill	Cadaver	Box trainers	Anatomic bench models	VR simulators
Precise portal placement	~	−	+	−
Triangulating the tip of the probe with a 30° scope	+	+	+	+
Insertion of the arthroscope	+	−	+	−
Entry of all compartments (medal/lateral/ posteromedial, suprapatellar/intercondylar)	+	−	+	+
Identification of all relevant structures in the knee joint (medial compartment, intercondylar notch, lateral compartment, lateral gutter, medial gutter)	+	−	+	+

Table 9.2 Crosstab within the left column the nine general requirements for simulator design and in the top row different types of simulators

General requirement	Cadaver	Box trainers	Anatomic bench models	VR simulators
Providing feedback	~	~	~	+
Repetitive practice	~	+	+	+
Curriculum integration	−	+	+	+
Range of difficulty level	~	−	~	+
Multiple learning strategies	−	~	~	~
Capture clinical variation	~	−	~	~
Controlled environment	−	+	+	+
Individualised learning	+	+	+	+
Defined outcomes	+	+	+	+

Additionally, the level of difficulty or availability of clinical variation cannot be preset per cadaver. When training on multiple cadavers, of course natural variation is available in size and anatomic structures but is more difficult to simulate different pathologies. In many countries, legislation is restrictive and prevents easy access to cadaver specimens, and if procured the cost of these specimens can be extremely high. Finally, cadavers require considerable preparation, especially when sensors are added to register training performance with defined outcomes and to offer feedback, objectively. Therefore, this type of training environment is less suitable for curriculum integration where training on a frequent repetitive basis is required. However, it can be very useful for advanced arthroscopists who are learning or developing new techniques or preparing for a rare but complex operation.

Box trainers are by definition low-fidelity trainers, which immediately indicates their limitation in offering different difficulty levels and clinical variation (Table 9.2). Their strengths are that they offer endless repetition in a highly controlled environment, which is convenient for novice residents as they truly focus on the basics and are allowed to make as many mistakes as needed. Provision of feedback can be offered by adding sensors in the box to register training performance with defined outcome measures.

Both anatomic bench models and virtual reality simulators possess all the general simulator requirements to a certain extent (Table 9.2). Anatomic bench models represent human joints. Some companies offer knee joints in different sizes and in a left and right version (Chap. 6), but similar to cadavers, this is not truly offering clinical variation in one model. The level of difficulty based on joint geometry cannot be changed, and most feedback that is given by residents indicates that the intra-articular joint space is unrealistically large, which compromises training when trainees have established basic arthroscopic skills proficiency. Some anatomic bench models do offer the possibility to simulate a bleeding, which increases complexity. Additionally, lots of different meniscal tears are usually available for training.

Again sensors can be added to the system to register performance. However, for all three training environments (cadavers, box trainers and anatomic bench models), it is noted that solely providing sensors is insufficient to offer supervisor-independent learning, as novices need to be guided in each step.

This latter aspect is the strength of virtual reality simulators. As these simulators are inherently computer based, they offer intuitive use of pictures, movies and other multimedia tools to support autonomous learning when using a simulator (Hurmusiadis et al. 2011; Megali et al. 2005). Additionally, as mathematical calculations are necessary anyhow to represent the virtual environment, metrics such as task time, path length and the number of unallowed tissue collisions can be easily documented and used for feedback and training progression. Finally, the level of clinical variation in the sense of different pathologies that can be trained is often abundant, but again most virtual reality simulators use only one knee configuration to train in.

9.5   Validation

Validation studies of the simulators are described in Chaps. 6 and 7 by searching literature databases (Pubmed and Scopus) using the following keywords: simulator name, 'arthroscopic simulator' and validity. Several authors recently have presented quite elegant overviews of the current

status of arthroscopic simulators, and in this section we will follow their work (Frank et al. 2014; Modi et al. 2010; Slade Shantz et al. 2014). The definitions of the different types of validity are described in Chap. 8.

9.5.1   Learning Curve

Learning curves are determined to demonstrate that there is training progression of the trainee (Table 9.3). The possibility of repetitive training is ranked in the top 10 of simulator requirements (Table 9.2) (Issenberg et al. 2005). All simulator environments qualify this requirement accept cadaver material. Howells and co-workers (Howells et al. 2009) clearly show the need for repetitive training. Unfortunately, repetitive performance of a task on a simulator does not indicate that the correct skills are trained. That is why testing of other types of validity is required, as we all know that having to relearn skills after incorrect training is harder than learning new skills.

9.5.2   Face Validity

Table 9.4 presents all studies that have tested the face validity of various simulators. Four out of the six are virtual reality simulators. Face validity testing is relatively easy to achieve as it merely requires a questionnaire and a group of experts indicating their opinion on the 'looks' of the simulator (e.g. Appendix 9.A). Despite this, it is not the most evaluated type of validity. This might be

Table 9.3 The learning curves as assessed after repeated training on various systems

Simulator	Type	Joint	Study
Procedicus™	VR simulator	Knee	Bliss et al. (2005)
Procedicus™	VR simulator	Shoulder	Gomoll et al. (2008)
SKATS	VR simulator	Knee	McCarthy et al. (2006), Moody et al. (2008)
Sawbones™	Anatomic bench model	Knee	Howells et al. (2008b), Jackson et al. (2012)
Sawbones™	Anatomic bench model	Shoulder	Howells et al. (2009)
Sawbones™	Anatomic bench model	Hip	Pollard et al. (2012)
Knee Arthroscopy Simulator	Anatomic bench model	Knee	Escoto et al. (2013)

Only papers are included that explicitly indicate the presence of a learning curve

Table 9.4 Inventory of all simulators that were tested for face validity

Simulator	Type	Joint	Study
SKATS	VR simulator	Knee	McCarthy and Hollands (1998), McCarthy et al. (2006), Moody et al. (2008)
Procedicus™	VR simulator	Shoulder	Srivastava et al. (2004)
Arthro Mentor™ (InsightArthroVR1)	VR simulator	Knee	Bayona et al. (2008), Tuijthof et al. (2011)
PASSPORT	Anatomic bench model	Knee	Tuijthof et al. (2010a), Tuijthof et al. (2012)
ArthroStim™	VR simulator	Knee	Tuijthof et al. (2011)
Knee Arthroscopy Simulator	Anatomic bench model	Knee	Escoto et al. (2013)

Only papers are included that explicitly indicate evaluation of face validity

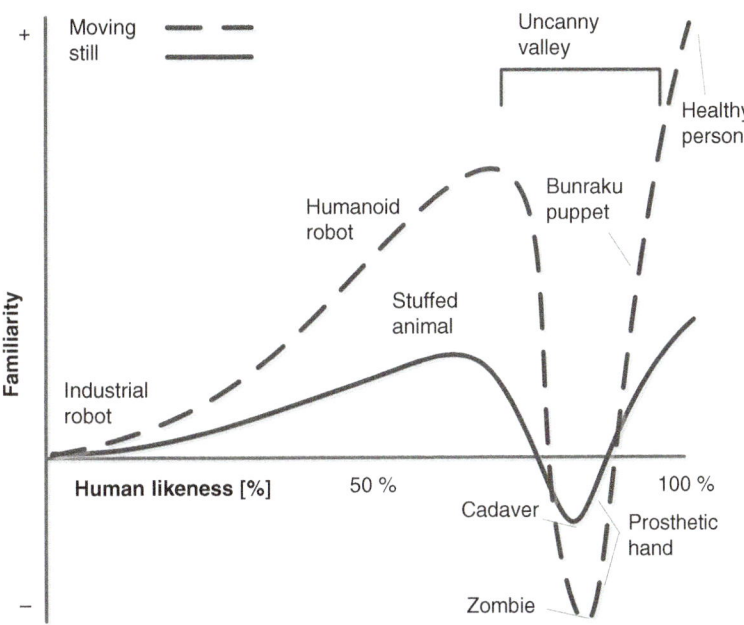

Fig. 9.1 Graphical illustration of the nonlinear relationship between the experience of negative and positive affect and perceived human likeness. The uncanny valley indicates the negative perceived realism even though the human-like object is highly realistic (Cheetham and Jancke 2013)

caused by the fact that simulator companies team up with a few experts surgeons when developing their systems and use those expert opinions to verify sufficient face validity. From a scientific point of view, questioning a larger panel of experts who are not directly involved in the development would provide stronger evidence.

Two other aspects need to be discussed regarding assessment of face validity. The first is the so-called *uncanny valley* effect (Cheetham and Jancke 2013; MacDorman 2005). The 'uncanny valley' hypothesis proposes that the perception of human-like characters such as robots or computer-generated avatars can evoke negative or positive affect depending on the object's degree of visual and behavioural realism along a dimension of human likeness (Fig. 9.1).

Although arthroscopic simulators are not human-like robots, they aim to represent part of the human. Even though we cannot provide scientific evidence, we noticed during our face validity tests that participants tend to become stricter in their judgment regarding the realism of a simulator, if that simulator has a high degree of realism. Contrary, the participants were more forgiving regarding simulators that clearly present a less realistic simulation of the human joint. Also, it should be taken into account that with current development in graphics of computer games, participants also increase their standards

Table 9.5 Inventory of all simulators that were tested for content validity

Simulator	Type	Joint	Study
Navigation Training Module	VR simulator	Knee	Megali et al. (2002), Megali et al. (2005)
Sawbones™	Anatomic bench model	Shoulder	Ceponis et al. (2007)
Arthro Mentor™ (InsightArthroVR1)	VR simulator	Knee	Bayona et al. (2008)

Only papers are included that explicitly indicate evaluation of content validity

regarding virtual reality simulation, as they know what could be possible. This suggests that the face validity judgment scale is nonlinear.

The second aspect that should be taken into account when interpreting face validity studies is the required realism of a simulator for the intended training purpose. This is nicely illustrated by Buzink and co-workers (Buzink et al. 2010) who showed that certain basic skills might be more efficiently trained in a truly abstract environment (such as a box trainer) than in an *almost realistic* virtual reality environment of a body part.

9.5.3   Content Validity

Table 9.5 presents all studies that have tested the content validity of various simulators. Noticeable are the short list of simulators and the fact that one of those is an anatomic bench model, which by itself has no means displaying the task to be trained. Two trends can be distinguished regarding the absence of numerous content validity testing presented in literature. Firstly, companies either develop tasks or exercises in close collaboration with a small group of experts or leave it to the ones that purchase their products to design their own tasks. Secondly, researchers who develop new concepts for simulated environments focus usually on one navigation task to indicate the proper performance of their system. In all, this properly reflects the fact that the execution of arthroscopic procedures can be performed in various ways. Therefore, this approach is suitable for informative training. However, if the future perspective is that summative training tests are going to be performed to demonstrate proficiency levels, it is highly recommended that

the arthroscopic community develops a set of validated tasks that can be used. This is not a trivial task, as it requires the decomposition of tasks into core steps. For expert surgeons that are so used to performing arthroscopy as, for example, riding a bike or tying shoe laces, it can be difficult to describe what they do and to distinguish between the various sequential actions.

9.5.4   Construct Validity

Table 9.6 presents all studies that have tested the construct validity of various simulators. Construct validity has been tested most extensively for both anatomic bench models and virtual reality simulators. All studies confirm construct validity between novices and experts, and this has been nicely presented by Slade Shantz and co-workers (2014).

Slade Shantz et al. 2014 in their recent systematic review. However, some critical remarks should be made (Modi et al. 2010; Slade Shantz et al. 2014): usually only one task is used (e.g. navigation and probe task), groups are small, levels of expertise are differently defined, and no evidence was found between intermediate and expert or novice groups. The latter could be explained by the fact that the intermediate group is the most heterogeneous group, and their motivation is possibly lowest (Srivastava et al. 2004; Tuijthof et al. 2011).

9.5.5   Concurrent Validity

Table 9.7 presents all studies that have tested the concurrent validity of various simulators. Concurrent validity is indirectly related to the performance of a simulator, as it concerns

Table 9.6 Inventory of all simulators that were tested for construct validity

Simulator	Type	Joint	Study
Procedicus™	VR simulator	Shoulder	Smith et al. (1999), Pedowitz et al. (2002), Srivastava et al. (2004), Gomoll et al. (2007), Gomoll et al. (2008)
VE-KATS	VR simulator	Knee	(Sherman et al. 2001)
SKATS	VR simulator	Knee	McCarthy et al. (2006), Moody et al. (2008)
Arthro Mentor™ (InsightArthroVR1)	VR simulator	Knee	Bayona et al. (2008), Tuijthof et al. (2011)
Arthro Mentor™ (InsightArthroVR1)	VR simulator	Shoulder	Andersen et al. (2011), Martin et al. (2012)
Sawbones™	Anatomic bench model	Shoulder	Howells et al. (2008a)
Sawbones™	Anatomic bench model	Knee	Tashiro et al. (2009)
PASSPORT	Anatomic bench model	Knee	Tuijthof et al. (2010a), Tuijthof et al. (2012)
Simendo Arthroscopy™	VR simulator	Knee	Tuijthof et al. (2010b)
ArthroStim™	VR simulator	Knee	Tuijthof et al. (2011), Cannon et al. (2014)
Human	Cadaver	Knee	Olson et al. (2013)

Only papers are included that explicitly indicate evaluation of construct validity

Table 9.7 Inventory of all simulators that were tested for concurrent validity

Simulator	Type	Joint	Study
Procedicus™	VR simulator	Shoulder	Smith et al. (1999), Pedowitz et al. (2002), Srivastava et al. (2004), Gomoll et al. (2007), Gomoll et al. (2008)
SKATS	VR simulator	Knee	McCarthy et al. (2006), Moody et al. (2008)
Sawbones™	Anatomic bench model	Shoulder	Howells et al. (2008a)
Sawbones™	Anatomic bench model	Knee	Tashiro et al. (2009)
Arthro Mentor™ (InsightArthroVR1)	VR simulator	Shoulder	Andersen et al. (2011)

Only papers are included that explicitly indicate evaluation of concurrent validity

the type of metrics that are used to indicate trainee performance. The studies that do measure multiple metrics usually track the task time, the path length and number of tissue collisions, which demonstrate a high correlation. In Chap. 11, many more potential metrics are described that could contribute to an overall performance profile of a trainee by combining efficiency and safety metrics.

9.5.6 Predictive or Transfer Validity

Table 9.8 presents all studies that have tested the predictive or transfer validity of various simulators. Predictive and transfer validity provide the most highest level of validity by indicating that

training of the simulated task transfers to actual performance in the operating room (Chap. 8). All but one of the studies presented in Table 9.8 present transfer validity to cadaver training, which is considered the preferred training modality of the surgeons (Chap. 2) (Safir et al. 2008; Vitale et al. 2007). Moody and co-workers studied transfer validity from one version of their SKAT simulator to an upgraded version in which passive haptic feedback was included (Moody et al. 2008). Only the study by Howells and co-workers (Howells et al. 2008b) demonstrates transfer validity to actual performance in the operating room. For their study, they used an anatomic bench model added with registration devices, which as demonstrated by them indicates a viable way of training.

Table 9.8 Inventory of all simulators that were tested for predictive or transfer validity

Validity	Simulator	Type	Joint	Study
Predictive	SKATS	VR simulator	Knee	McCarthy et al. (2006)
Transfer	SKATS	VR simulator	Knee	Moody et al. (2008)
Transfer	Sawbones™	Anatomic bench model	Knee	Howells et al. (2008b), Butler et al. (2013)
Transfer	Arthro Mentor™ (InsightArthroVR1)	VR simulator	Shoulder	Martin et al. (2011)
Transfer	Procedicus™	VR simulator	Shoulder	Henn III et al. (2013)

Only papers are included that explicitly indicate evaluation of predictive or transfer validity

9.6 Case Example Standardised Study Protocol

Modi and co-workers (Modi et al. 2010) indicated a range of limitations on the methodology used in evaluation studies of simulators: the use of poorly validated outcome measures, the absence of multiple centre studies and the impossibility of comparing groups or simulators. In an effort to overcome a number of these limitations, we have set up a general study protocol to assess face and construct validity of any type of arthroscopic simulators (Tuijthof et al. 2011). This protocol enables evaluation and relative comparison of any type of simulator (virtual reality or phantom). We have evaluated ArthroStim™ (Touch of Life Technologies, Aurora, CO, USA: Simulator A), Arthro Mentor™ (Simbionix, Cleveland, Ohio, USA, previously known as the InsightArthroVR1 Arthroscopy Simulator (GMV, Madrid, Spain): Simulator B), VirtaMed ArthroS™ (VirtaMed AG, Zurich, Switzerland: Simulator D) and our own development the PASSPORT simulator (Delft University of Technology and Academic Medical Centre, The Netherlands: Simulator C). In short the protocol is set up as follows.

Participants were recruited and grouped in different experience levels. Only the results are presented of novices who had never performed an arthroscopic procedure and experts who had performed more than 60 arthroscopies. The level of 60 was set using a study by O'Neill and co-workers (O'Neill et al. 2002) who questioned a large group of fellow ship directors who indi-

cated a mean of 62 arthroscopies to be performed in other to achieve proficiency. Between 6 and 11 participants were present in each experience group for each simulator. All participants were scheduled a maximum period of 30 min in order to be able to recruit experts.

Face validity, educational value and user-friendliness of the simulators were determined by the participants performing up to three exercise(s) that were characteristic for that particular simulator. Clear instructions were given that performance of these exercises would not be documented, and the researcher pointed explicitly to manner in which performance feedback was given to the participant. Afterwards the participants were asked to fill out a questionnaire (Appendix 9.A) (Tuijthof et al. 2011). Questions were answered using a 10-point numerical rating scale (NRS) (e.g. 0=completely unrealistic and 10=completely realistic). Only the answers of the intermediates and experts regarding face validity and educational value were included. A value of 7 or greater was considered as being satisfactory. Face validity of the outer appearance was demonstrated for all simulators, but only simulator C demonstrated face validity for intra-articular joint realism and instrument realism (Fig. 9.2). This result was significantly different from simulator B for intra-articular joint realism and significantly different from all simulators for instrument realism ($p < 0.05$). The explanation is that simulator C is the only system that uses real instruments and a knee bench-top model to mimic sense of touch, which was considered

Fig. 9.2 Face validity and user-friendliness of four simulators

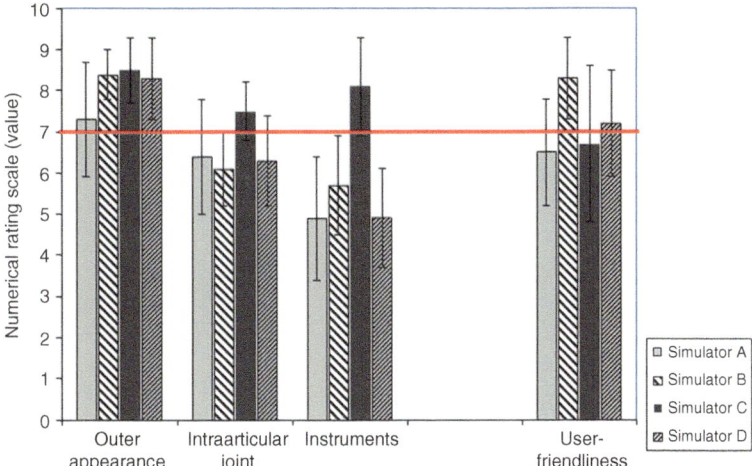

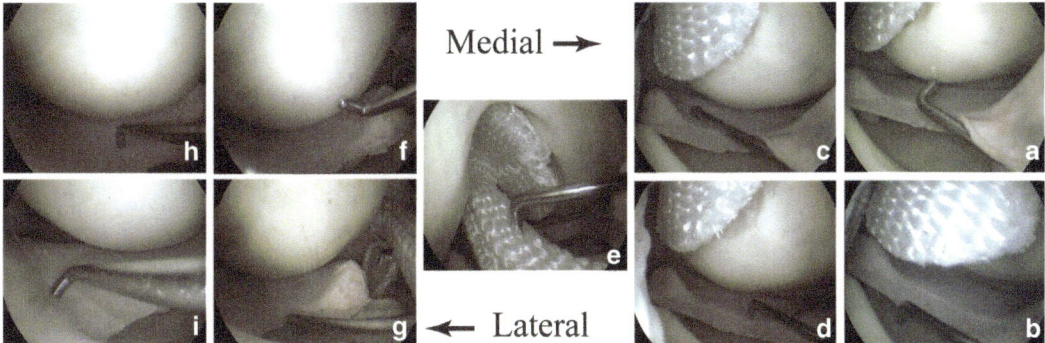

Fig. 9.3 Pictures of the intra-articular joint space of simulator C. The landmarks had to be probed in the following sequence for the navigation task: (**a**) medial femoral condyle, (**b**) medial tibial plateau, (**c**) posterior horn of medial meniscus, (**d**) midsection of medial meniscus, (**e**) anterior cruciate ligament, (**f**) lateral femoral condyle, (**g**) lateral tibial plateau, (**h**) posterior horn of lateral meniscus and (**i**) midsection of lateral meniscus (© GJM Tuijthof, 2014. Reprinted with permission)

the biggest asset by the participants. Simulators B and D demonstrate good user-friendliness, with the difference between simulators A and B being significant ($p < 0.05$). All virtual reality simulators needed improvement of the sense of touch. All simulators could benefit from more realistic structures but were considered as valuable training tool in the beginning of the residency curriculum.

Construct validity was assessed based on a single predefined navigation task. Nine anatomic landmarks had to be probed sequentially: medial femoral condyle, medial tibial plateau, posterior horn of the medial meniscus, midsection of the medial meniscus, ACL, lateral femoral condyle, lateral tibial plateau, posterior horn of the lateral meniscus and midsection of the lateral meniscus (Fig. 9.3) (Tuijthof et al. 2010a). The task trial times were recorded by separate digital video recording equipment to guarantee uniformity in data processing. All participants performed the navigation task 5 times. Construct validity was determined with the Kruskal–Wallis test by calculation of overall significant differences in task time between the three groups for each of the five task trials.

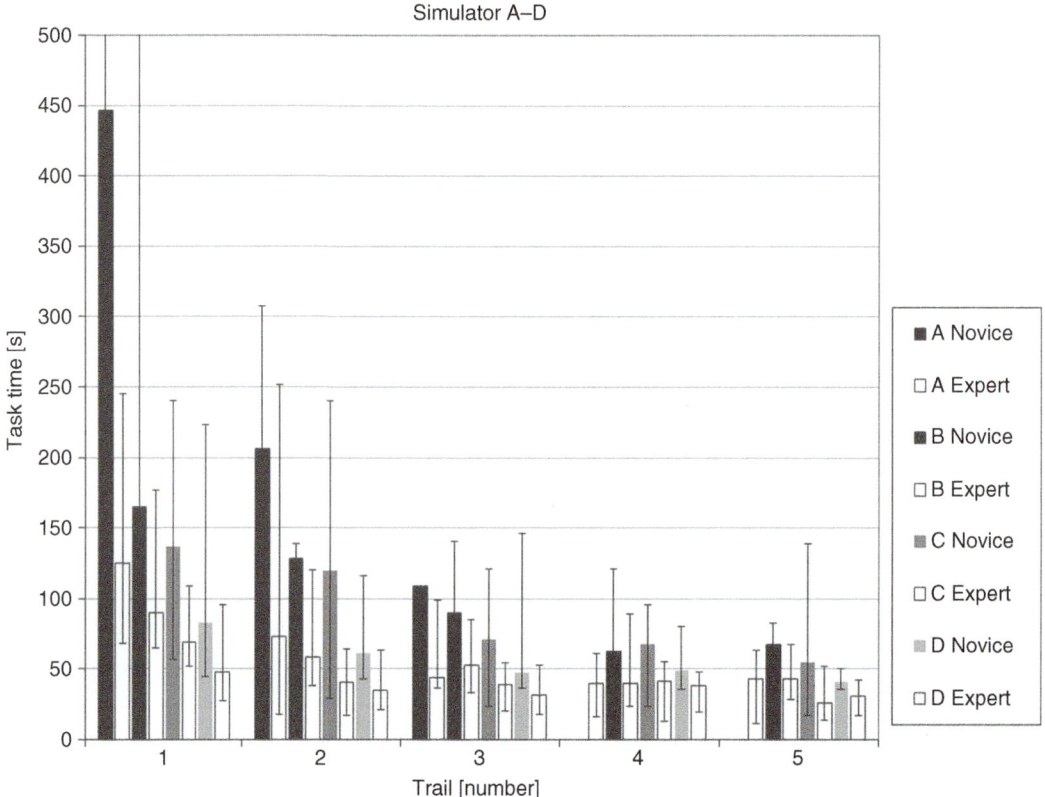

Fig. 9.4 Construct validity of four simulators

The significance level was adjusted for multiple comparisons with the Bonferroni–Holm procedure (alpha = 0.05) (Holm 1979). Mann–Whitney U tests were used for pair-wise comparisons to highlight significant differences. Construct validity was shown for simulators C and D, as the novices were significantly slower than the experts in completing all five trials (Fig. 9.4). For simulator A, only 2 out of 11 novices could complete all task trials within the set time limit. This indicates a clear distinction between novices and experts, which unfortunately cannot be supported by actual measurements. Simulator B partly demonstrated construct validity as the experts were faster in the second and third trials compared to the novices.

As the same navigation and probe task were performed on all simulators, it allows comparison of the performance of the experts. All expert task times of trial 5 are in the same range, and do not significantly differ. This suggests that for the evaluated navigation task, training on any of the simulators yields the same performance results. A noticeable distinction between the learning curves of the experts is that simulator A shows a steep learning curve with trial 1 being significantly slower than trial 5, while simulator D shows no significant difference between trials 1 and 5.

This might suggest that the virtual reality environment of simulator D is the most realistic as experts do not have to become acquainted with the simulator.

9.7 Discussion

Analysing the wishes from the arthroscopic community, the conclusion is that triangulating the tip of the probe with a 30° scope, entry of all compartments and identification of all relevant structures in the knee joint can be trained with currently available arthroscopic simulators (Table 9.1). Precise portal placement and adequate insertion of the arthroscope cannot be trained. As indicated in Chap. 6, efforts are being made to enhance skin realism and allow repetitive training of portal placement.

Analysing the general requirements regarding simulator design, both anatomic bench models and virtual reality simulators possess all general simulator requirements to a certain extent (Table 9.2). They therefore appear to be most suitable for integration in a training curriculum. Notice that for objective performance tracking and autonomous training, anatomic bench models need to be complemented with registration devices and multimedia tools. On the other hand, virtual reality simulators need improvement regarding haptic feedback (Moody et al. 2008; Tuijthof et al. 2010a; Zivanovic et al. 2003). Both box trainers and cadaver training have limitations, which makes them more suitable for training in a distinct part of the entire training process: at the very beginning of the learning curve (box trainers) and at the end of the learning curve, where experienced arthroscopists want to learn a new technique or a difficult procedure (cadaver material).

Validation tests have been performed by the pioneers in the late 1990s and early zeros.

They developed virtual reality simulators by applying new computer science techniques or used conventional anatomic bench model to demonstrate effect of training outside the operating room (Bliss et al. 2005; McCarthy and Hollands 1998; Megali et al. 2002; Pedowitz et al. 2002; Sherman et al. 2001; Smith et al. 1999; Srivastava et al. 2004). It is worth noting that it was simulators of the knee and shoulder joint that were evaluated. Unfortunately some of the simulators that have been quite extensively validated (Procedicus™ shoulder joint) are no longer commercially available or have never been further developed into a commercial product (SKATS and PASSPORT knee joint simulators) (Tables 9.3, 9.4, 9.5, 9.6, 9.7, and 9.8). However, including those simulators in this chapter helps provide a strong indication that, similarly in other endoscopic fields, arthroscopic simulators demonstrate face and construct validity (Slade Shantz et al. 2014) and to some extent content, concurrent and transfer validity. Additionally, training in a simulated environment correlates to improved skill (Frank et al. 2014; Modi et al. 2010), which ultimately should increase patient safety and efficiency in training time.

There is however still scope for improving validation studies as stated by Modi and coworkers (Modi et al. 2010): the use of validated outcome measures, multiple centre studies, study designs that allow group and simulator comparison and assessment of transfer validity are all areas that still need research and development.

Appendix 9.A Questionnaire Face Validity and Usability

The questionnaire will remain anonymous! Please fill in all the questions by encircling one number ranging from 0 to 10, much as you would score an exam. Encircling *N/A* if the question does not apply to you. Encircling one of the options that applies to you and filling in the boxes if needed.

General questions

What is your age?

What is your gender?

Male   **Female**

How many arthroscopic surgeries of the knee did you perform?

0*   **1 - 59**   **> 60**

*If answered 0, how many arthroscopic surgeries have you witnessed last year?

Did you previously have arthroscopy training sessions with one or more of the following modalities? *(more than one option is allowed)*

No   **cadaveric material**   **virtual reality simulator***   **physical phantom***

*Please specify product name:

Do you have experience in playing computer games?

Yes*	No

*If answered yes, please specify the hours per week and for how many years:

Hours per week	Years

Questions regarding the simulator before evaluation test

What is your opinion on the outer appearance of <u>any</u> simulator?

Not important, the intra-articular anatomy is what matters	Important, the joint should be directly recognizable on the outside

What is your opinion on the outer appearance of <u>this</u> simulator?

Complete-ly unrealistic	0	1	2	3	4	5	6	7	8	9	10	Completely realistic

Is it clear in which joint you will be operating?

Complete-ly unclear	0	1	2	3	4	5	6	7	8	9	10	Completely clear

Questions regarding the simulator after evaluation test

Questions concerning the realism of the simulator

The not applicable (N/A) option is only allowed if you have not performed any arthroscopic operations or have seen less than 5 arthroscopic operations.

Is it clear which portals are being used?   N/A

| Complete-ly unclear | 0 | 1 | 2 | 3 | 4 | 5 | 6 | 7 | 8 | 9 | 1 0 | Com-pletely clear |

How realistic is the intra-articular anatomy?   N/A

| Complete-ly unreal-istic | 0 | 1 | 2 | 3 | 4 | 5 | 6 | 7 | 8 | 9 | 1 0 | Com-pletely realistic |

Are all essential anatomic structures present?

| Yes | No* | N/A |

*If answered with no, which structure(s) do you miss?

How realistic is the texture of the structures?   N/A

Complete-ly unreal-istic	0	1	2	3	4	5	6	7	8	9	10	Com-pletely realistic

How realistic is the color of the structures?   N/A

Complete-ly unreal-istic	0	1	2	3	4	5	6	7	8	9	10	Com-pletely realistic

How realistic is the size of the structures?   N/A

Complete-ly unreal-istic	0	1	2	3	4	5	6	7	8	9	10	Com-pletely realistic

How realistic is the size of the intra-articular joint space?   N/A

Complete-ly unreal-istic	0	1	2	3	4	5	6	7	8	9	10	Com-pletely realistic

How realistic is the arthroscopic image itself?   N/A

Complete-ly unreal-istic	0	1	2	3	4	5	6	7	8	9	10	Com-pletely realistic

Questions concerning the instruments

Is it clear what instruments you are using?

Yes	No	N/A

How realistic do the instruments look?   N/A

Complete-ly unrealistic	0	1	2	3	4	5	6	7	8	9	10	Completely realistic

How realistic is the motion of your instruments?   N/A

Complete-ly unrealistic	0	1	2	3	4	5	6	7	8	9	10	Completely realistic

Is there any delay between the movements you make and those projected on-screen?

Yes	No	N/A

How realistic does the tissue feel when you are probing?   N/A

Complete-ly unrealistic	0	1	2	3	4	5	6	7	8	9	10	Completely realistic

How realistic does the tissue feel when you are cutting?   N/A

Complete-ly unrealistic	0	1	2	3	4	5	6	7	8	9	10	Completely realistic

Questions concerning usage

How clear are the instructions to start an exercise on the simulator?

Complete-ly unclear	0	1	2	3	4	5	6	7	8	9	1 0	**Com-pletely clear**

Did you feel the need to read a manual before operating the simulator?

Yes	**No**

How do you feel about the variation in exercises offered by the simulator?

Too little	**Adequate**	**Too much**

How do you feel about the difference in required skill level between exercises?

Too little	**Adequate**	**Too much**

If the virtual reality environment does not represent a joint, are the exercises still suitable to train arthroscopic skills?

Yes	**No**	**N/A**

Does the simulator allow training of joint inspection?

Yes	**No**

Does the simulator allow training of joint irrigation?

Yes	**No**

Does the simulator allow therapeutic interventions?

Yes	No

How clear is the presentation of your performance by the simulator?

Complete-ly unreal-istic	0	1	2	3	4	5	6	7	8	9	1 0	Com-pletely realistic

Is it clear how you can improve your performance?

Complete-ly unreal-istic	0	1	2	3	4	5	6	7	8	9	1 0	Com-pletely realistic

How motivating is the way the results are presented to improve your performance?

Most de-motivat-ing	0	1	2	3	4	5	6	7	8	9	1 0	Most mo-tivating

Question concerning educational value

Do you think the simulator is a suitable training modality in a skills-lab?
N/A

Most un-suited	0	1	2	3	4	5	6	7	8	9	1 0	Most suited

Do you think using this simulator is a good way to prepare for a real-life arthroscopic operation?

Yes*   No*

*Please specify your answer:

 At what stage in the residency curriculum do you think the simulator will be most valuable as a training modality?

Suggestions / Improvements

Please mention at least two points

End of questionnaire. Thank you very much for your cooperation!

Bibliography

Andersen C, Winding TN, Vesterby MS (2011) Development of simulated arthroscopic skills. Acta Orthop 82(1):90–95, available from: PM:21281257

Bayona S, Fernandez-Arroyo JM, Martin I, Bayona P (2008) Assessment study of insightARTHRO VR arthroscopy virtual training simulator: face, content, and construct validities. J Robotic Surg 2(3):151–158

Bliss JP, Hanner-Bailey HS, Scerbo MW (2005) Determining the efficacy of an immersive trainer for arthroscopic skills. Stud Health Technol Inform 111:54–56, available from: PM:15718698

Butler A, Olson T, Koehler R, Nicandri G (2013) Do the skills acquired by novice surgeons using anatomic dry models transfer effectively to the task of diagnostic knee arthroscopy performed on cadaveric specimens? J Bone Joint Surg Am 95(3):e15–e18, available from: PM:23389795

Buzink SN, Christie LS, Goossens RH, de Ridder H, Jakimowicz JJ (2010) Influence of anatomic landmarks in the virtual environment on simulated angled laparoscope navigation. Surg Endosc 24(12):2993–3001, available from: PM:20419318

Cannon WD, Nicandri GT, Reinig K, Mevis H, Wittstein J (2014) Evaluation of skill level between trainees and community orthopaedic surgeons using a virtual reality arthroscopic knee simulator. J Bone Joint Surg Am 96(7):e57, available from: PM:24695934

Ceponis PJ, Chan D, Boorman RS, Hutchison C, Mohtadi NG (2007) A randomized pilot validation of educational measures in teaching shoulder arthroscopy to surgical residents. Can J Surg 50(5):387–393, available from: PM:18031640

Cheetham M, Jancke L (2013) Perceptual and category processing of the Uncanny Valley hypothesis' dimension of human likeness: some methodological issues. J Vis Exp 76:1–15, available from: PM:23770728

Escoto A, Le BF, Trejos AL, Naish MD, Patel RV, Lebel ME (2013) A knee arthroscopy simulator: design and validation. Conf Proc IEEE Eng Med Biol Soc 2013:5715–5718, available from: PM:24111035

Frank RM, Erickson B, Frank JM, Bush-Joseph CA, Bach BR Jr, Cole BJ, Romeo AA, Provencher MT, Verma NN (2014) Utility of modern arthroscopic simulator training models. Arthroscopy 30(1):121–133, available from: PM:24290789

Gomoll AH, O'Toole RV, Czarnecki J, Warner JJ (2007) Surgical experience correlates with performance on a virtual reality simulator for shoulder arthroscopy. Am J Sports Med 35(6):883–888, available from: PM:17261572

Gomoll AH, Pappas G, Forsythe B, Warner JJ (2008) Individual skill progression on a virtual reality simulator for shoulder arthroscopy: a 3-year follow-up study. Am J Sports Med 36(6):1139–1142, available from: PM:18326032

Henn RF III, Shah N, Warner JJ, Gomoll AH (2013) Shoulder arthroscopy simulator training improves shoulder arthroscopy performance in a cadaveric model. Arthroscopy 29(6):982–985, available from: PM:23591380

Holm S (1979) A simple sequentially rejective multiple test procedure. Scand J Stat 6(2):65–70

Howells NR, Auplish S, Hand GC, Gill HS, Carr AJ, Rees JL (2009) Retention of arthroscopic shoulder skills learned with use of a simulator. Demonstration of a learning curve and loss of performance level after a time delay. J Bone Joint Surg Am 91(5):1207–1213, available from: PM:19411470

Howells NR, Brinsden MD, Gill RS, Carr AJ, Rees JL (2008a) Motion analysis: a validated method for showing skill levels in arthroscopy. Arthroscopy 24(3):335–342, available from: PM:18308187

Howells NR, Gill HS, Carr AJ, Price AJ, Rees JL (2008b) Transferring simulated arthroscopic skills to the operating theatre: a randomised blinded study. J Bone Joint Surg Br 90(4):494–499, available from: PM:18378926

Hurmusiadis V, Rhode K, Schaeffter T, Sherman K (2011) Virtual arthroscopy trainer for minimally invasive surgery. Stud Health Technol Inform 163:236–238, available from: PM:21335795

Issenberg SB, McGaghie WC, Petrusa ER, Lee GD, Scalese RJ (2005) Features and uses of high-fidelity medical simulations that lead to effective learning: a BEME systematic review. Med Teach 27(1):10–28, available from: PM:16147767

Jackson WF, Khan T, Alvand A, Al-Ali S, Gill HS, Price AJ, Rees JL (2012) Learning and retaining simulated arthroscopic meniscal repair skills. J Bone Joint Surg Am 94(17):e132, available from: PM:22992861

MacDorman K. Androids as an experimental apparatus: why is there an uncanny valley and can we exploit it? In: Toward Social Mechanisms of Android Science: A CogSci 2005 Workshop, pp 106–118

Martin KD, Belmont PJ, Schoenfeld AJ, Todd M, Cameron KL, Owens BD (2011) Arthroscopic basic task performance in shoulder simulator model correlates with similar task performance in cadavers. J Bone Joint Surg Am 93(21):e1271–e1275, available from: PM:22048106

Martin KD, Cameron K, Belmont PJ, Schoenfeld A, Owens BD (2012) Shoulder arthroscopy simulator performance correlates with resident and shoulder arthroscopy experience. J Bone Joint Surg Am 94(21):e160, available from: PM:23138247

McCarthy AD, Hollands RJ (1998) A commercially viable virtual reality knee arthroscopy training system. Stud Health Technol Inform 50:302–308, available from: PM:10180558

McCarthy AD, Moody L, Waterworth AR, Bickerstaff DR (2006) Passive haptics in a knee arthroscopy simulator: is it valid for core skills training? Clin Orthop Relat Res 442:13–20, available from: PM:16394733

McGaghie WC, Issenberg SB, Petrusa ER, Scalese RJ (2010) A critical review of simulation-based medical education research: 2003-2009. Med Educ 44(1):50–63, available from: PM:20078756

Megali G, Tonet O, Mazzoni M, Dario P, Vascellari A, Marcacci M (2002) Proc of the 5th Int. Conf. on Medical Image Computing and Computer-assisted intervention part II, A new tool for surgical training in knee arthroscopy. In: Dohi T, Kikinis R (eds), Tokio, pp 170–177

Megali G, Tonet O, Dario P, Vascellari A, Marcacci M (2005) Computer-assisted training system for knee arthroscopy. Int J Med Robot 1(3):57–66, available from: PM:17518391

Modi CS, Morris G, Mukherjee R (2010) Computer-simulation training for knee and shoulder arthroscopic surgery. Arthroscopy 26(6):832–840, available from: PM:20511043

Moody L, Waterworth A, McCarthy AD, Harley P, Smallwood R (2008) The feasibility of a mixed reality surgical training environment. Virtual Real 12:77–86

O'Neill PJ, Cosgarea AJ, Freedman JA, Queale WS, McFarland EG (2002) Arthroscopic proficiency: a survey of orthopaedic sports medicine fellowship directors and orthopaedic surgery department chairs. Arthroscopy 18(7):795–800, available from: PM:12209439

Olson T, Koehler R, Butler A, Amsdell S, Nicandri G (2013) Is there a valid and reliable assessment of diagnostic knee arthroscopy skill? Clin Orthop Relat Res 471(5):1670–1676, available from: PM:23254692

Pedowitz RA, Esch J, Snyder S (2002) Evaluation of a virtual reality simulator for arthroscopy skills development. Arthroscopy 18(6):E29, available from: PM:12098111

Pollard TC, Khan T, Price AJ, Gill HS, Glyn-Jones S, Rees JL (2012) Simulated hip arthroscopy skills: learning curves with the lateral and supine patient positions: a randomized trial. J Bone Joint Surg Am 94(10):e68, available from: PM:22617934

Safir O, Dubrowski A, Mirsky L, Lin C, Backstein D, Carnahan A (2008) What skills should simulation training in arthroscopy teach residents? Int J Comp Assist Radiol Surg 3(5):433–437

Sherman KP, Ward JW, Wills DP, Sherman VJ, Mohsen AM (2001) Surgical trainee assessment using a VE knee arthroscopy training system (VE-KATS): experimental results. Stud Health Technol Inform 81:465–470, available from: PM:11317792

Slade Shantz JA, Leiter JR, Gottschalk T, MacDonald PB (2014) The internal validity of arthroscopic simulators and their effectiveness in arthroscopic education. Knee Surg SportsTraumatol Arthrosc 22(1):33–40, available from: PM:23052120

Smith S, Wan A, Taffinder N, Read S, Emery R, Darzi A (1999) Early experience and validation work with Procedicus V--he Prosolvia virtual reality shoulder arthroscopy trainer. Stud HealthTechnol Inform 62:337–343, available from: PM:10538383

Srivastava S, Youngblood PL, Rawn C, Hariri S, Heinrichs WL, Ladd AL (2004) Initial evaluation of a shoulder arthroscopy simulator: establishing construct validity. J Shoulder Elbow Surg 13(2):196–205, available from: PM:14997099

Stunt JJ, Kerkhoffs GM, Horeman T, van Dijk CN, Tuijthof GJM (2014) Validation of the PASSPORT V2 training environment for arthroscopic skills, Knee Surg Sports Traumatol Arthrosc, epub 8 Aug 2014 PM:25103120

Tashiro Y, Miura H, Nakanishi Y, Okazaki K, Iwamoto Y (2009) Evaluation of skills in arthroscopic training based on trajectory and force data. Clin Orthop Relat Res 467((2):546–552, available from: PM:18791774

Tuijthof GJ, van Sterkenburg MN, Sierevelt IN, Van OJ, van Dijk CN, Kerkhoffs GM (2010a) First validation of the PASSPORT training environment for arthroscopic skills. Knee Surg Sports Traumatol Arthrosc 18(2)):218–224, available from: PM:19629441

Tuijthof GJ, Visser P, Sierevelt IN, van Dijk CN, Kerkhoffs GM (2011) Does perception of usefulness of arthroscopic simulators differ with levels of experience? Clin Orthop Relat Res, available from: PM:21290203

Tuijthof G, Sierevelt IN, Dijk C, Kerkhoffs G (2010b) Is the presence of a dummy leg essential in the SIMENDO arthroscopy trainer? Knee Surg Sport Tr A 18(1):16

Ref Type: Abstract

Vitale MA, Kleweno CP, Jacir AM, Levine WN, Bigliani LU, Ahmad CS (2007) Training resources in arthroscopic rotator cuff repair. J Bone Joint Surg Am 89(6):1393–1398, available from: PM:17545443

Zivanovic A, Dibble E, Davies B, Moody L, Waterworth A (2003) Engineering requirements for a haptic simulator for knee arthroscopy training. Stud Health Technol Inform 94:413–418, available from: PM:15455938

Preclinical Training Strategies

10

Gabriëlle J.M. Tuijthof, Izaäk F. Kodde,
and Gino M.M.J. Kerkhoffs

*We believe that the use of simulation will shorten surgical training times
and helps to reduce surgical complications for the patients.*

Take-Home Messages

- Arthroscopic simulator training by surgical trainees improves technical performance in the operating theater.
- Interval practice is a more effective training schedule than massed practice.
- Residents can successfully teach in the skills laboratory, and their teaching skills are acceptable compared with those of faculty instructors.

10.1 Introduction

With innovations in the surgical training program, the need for alternative surgical skills training methods becomes more and more important. Over 80 % of orthopedic residents and orthopedic program directors in the USA agreed that surgical simulation should become a required part of orthopedic resident training. (Karam et al. 2013). However, surgical

G.J.M. Tuijthof (✉)
Department of Biomechanical Engineering,
Delft University of Technology, Delft,
The Netherlands

Department of Orthopedic Surgery,
Academic Medical Centre, Amsterdam,
The Netherlands
e-mail: g.j.m.tuijthof@tudelft.nl

I.F. Kodde • G.M.M.J. Kerkhoffs
Department of Orthopedic Surgery, Academic
Medical Centre, Amsterdam, The Netherlands
e-mail: i.f.kodde@amc.uva.nl;
g.m.kerkhoffs@amc.uva.nl

skills facilities were not available in almost 25 % of training sites. The main obstruction to create formal surgical skills programs was a lack of money (Karam et al. 2013). Karam and coworkers (Karam et al. 2013) therefore concluded that orthopedic educators should find cost-effective solutions to improve surgical skills training. This chapter describes different kinds of preclinical training strategies for orthopedic residents in arthroscopic surgery.

10.2 Simulators

The simulators used for training arthroscopic surgery can be classified into physical simulators, virtual reality simulators, and hybrid simulators (Fig. 10.1). Physical simulators include human or animal cadavers or artificial models. Virtual reality simulators are video based or computer based. Whenever virtual reality simulators are combined with physical components for real tactile feedback, these are named hybrid simulators (Madan and Pai 2014). All different types of stimulators are discussed in Chaps. 5, 6 and 7.

10.3 Factors Affecting Preclinical Skills Acquisition

10.3.1 Level of Experience

Several studies evaluated the ability of simulators to differentiate between novice and expert arthroscopic surgeons (Andersen et al. 2011; Pedowitz et al. 2002;

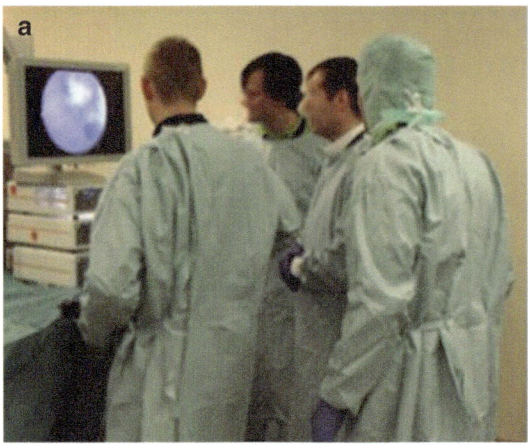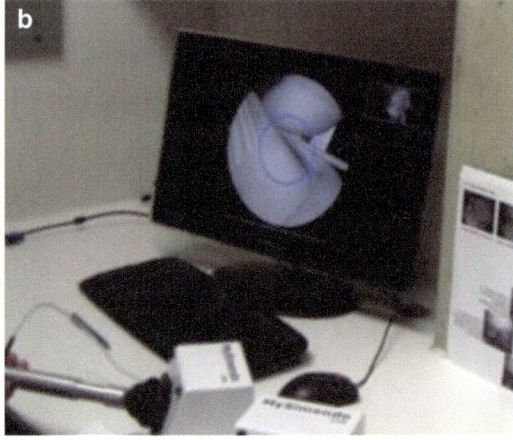

Fig. 10.1 Arthroscopic simulation training in practice (© I.F. Kodde, 2014. Reprinted with permission)

Tuijthof et al. 2010). All studies found good construct validity for virtual reality simulators, with experienced surgeons performing tasks faster and with more efficiency compared to residents and interns.

Interestingly, a 5-h training for inexperienced trainees on a virtual reality simulator was sufficient to perform better than the experienced surgeons in a second test (Andersen et al. 2011). So it is suggested that simulators provide the greatest performance gain for novice trainees (Madan and Pai 2014). The abovementioned results indicate that the simulator does show deviations from real arthroscopic surgery. However, the fact that experienced surgeons outperformed the inexperienced colleagues on a virtual reality simulator indicates that these skills are somewhat transferable. Furthermore, one RCT compared two groups of orthopedic trainees to investigate the transfer validity of arthroscopic skills from simulator to the operating theater. One group received a fixed protocol of simulator training before performance in the operating theater was assessed. The control group did not have simulator training before practice in the operating theater (such as in the traditional training schemes). The simulator-trained group significantly outscored the untrained group in terms of both the Orthopedic Competence Assessment Project and global rating scores (Appendix 13.A). Thus, arthroscopic simulator training by surgical trainees improves technical performance in the operating theater (Howells et al. 2008).

10.3.2 Video Games

Rosenthal and coworkers compared virtual reality task performance of children with different levels of experience in video games and residents. They concluded that the use of computer games may contribute to the development of skills relevant for adequate performance in laparoscopic virtual reality tasks (Rosenthal et al. 2011). However, others contradicted this theory (Harper et al. 2007; Thorson et al. 2011).

10.3.3 Innate Skills

The acquisition of a new surgical skill is characterized by a learning curve and the progress of an individual on the curve might be influenced by the innate ability of the individual to acquire a skill. It has been questioned whether variations in arthroscopic skills of trainees are caused by the training provided or rather by innate skills. Alvand and coworkers observed considerable variability in the arthroscopic ability of medical students and hypothesized that this was due to innate arthroscopic ability since none of the study subjects had any previous exposure to the tasks in question (Alvand et al. 2011). However, it has also been suggested that self-reported interest in surgery is a better predictor than innate skills for learning simulated arthroscopic surgery tasks (Madan and Pai 2014; Thorson et al. 2011).

10.3.4 Gender

Sex differences have been found to exist in the acquisition of skills (Strandbygaard et al. 2013). Thorson et al. evaluated laparoscopic skills among medical students and found that female students performed worse on the laparoscopic trainer than males after adjusting for age, choice of medical specialty, and video game use. They concluded that female medical students differ in their innate abilities on the laparoscopic trainer which might be related to a different psychomotor skill acquisition and behavior of females compared to males (Thorson et al. 2011).

10.3.5 Timing of Simulator Training

The acquisition of motor skills may be influenced by the time of day. Bonrath and coworkers evaluated whether results of laparoscopic training were different based on the time of day (morning, afternoon, or evening) the training was provided. There were no differences observed between the groups with training during working hours (morning and afternoon) and after working hours (evening). All participants significantly improved in laparoscopic skills (Bonrath et al. 2013). Rest appears to be an important adjunct to effective practice; more than four hours of practice per day causes the quality of practice to deteriorate and leads to fatigue. Also, an adequate amount of sleep seems to be a predictor of success on a laparoscopic surgery simulator (Wanzel et al. 2002). The acquisition of skills is also dependent on the training schedules. Practice sessions can be either a single long session (massed practice) or multiple short sessions (interval practice). It has been shown that interval practice is a more effective training schedule than massed practice. This has probably to do with the theory that the skills being learned have more time to be cognitively consolidated between practices (Gallagher et al. 2005).

10.3.6 Instructors

Strandbygaard and coworkers (Strandbygaard et al. 2013) performed a RCT to evaluate the feedback of an instructor during a virtual reality simulator course. Feedback was defined as the provision or return of performance-related information to the performer. Instructor feedback increased efficiency when training a complex operational task on a virtual reality simulator; time and repetitions used to achieve a predefined proficiency level were significantly reduced in the group that received instructor feedback compared with the control group. In addition, they found that the feedback influenced the females' performance more than that of males (Strandbygaard et al. 2013). However, in more basic tasks, such as coordination and instrument navigation, no specific advantages of instructor feedback have been found (Snyder et al. 2009). Also, it has been shown that residents can successfully teach in the skills laboratory and that their teaching skills are acceptable compared with faculty instructors (Pernar et al. 2012).

Conclusion
Simulation is being used more and more in arthroscopic training for the acquisition of both basic and advanced arthroscopic surgical skills. The impact of virtual reality training is currently more established in the field of laparoscopy rather than arthroscopy. While there are no comparative studies that evaluated whether the results of virtual reality in laparoscopy also account for arthroscopy, it is generally believed that the acquisition of basic skills such as coordination and instrument navigation will be comparable for the two. Although the consensus at the present still seems to be that simulators are useful in arthroscopic training but are adjuncts to real experience and cannot fully replace it, we believe that the use of simulation will shorten surgical training times and helps to reduce surgical complications for the patients. With the development of more sophisticated

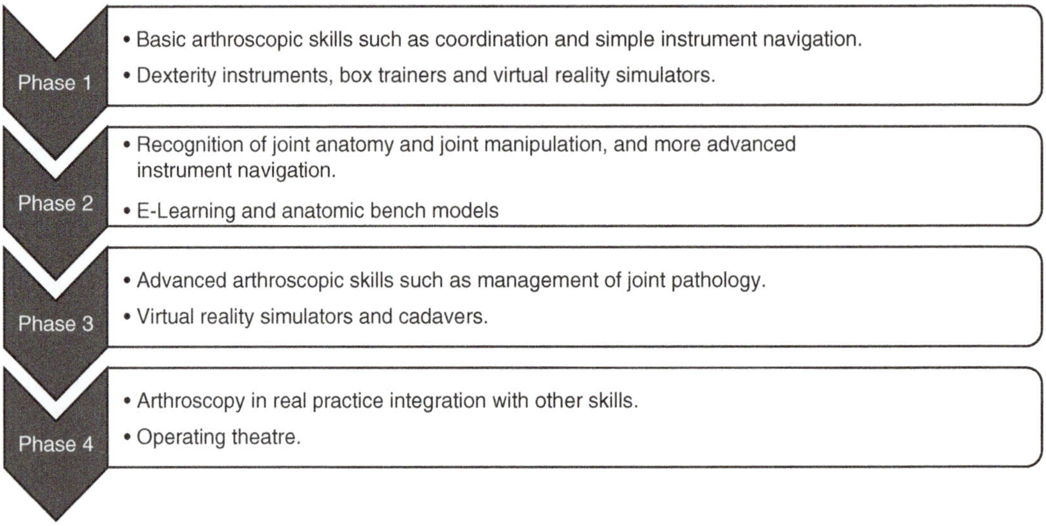

Fig. 10.2 Proposal for strategy to effectively train arthroscopic skills

simulators, it is likely that these will present an important part of future arthroscopic surgical training programs.

10.4 Approach for Arthroscopic Simulator Training

The success of preclinical simulator training depends on numerous factors. Based on the abovementioned factors, a 3-step approach for arthroscopic simulator training has been suggested by Madan and coworkers (Madan and Pai 2014). The first step would be to provide hand-eye coordination and simple manipulation training on box trainers. The second step would be to provide instrument navigations skills and recognition of joint anatomy. The third step would be to provide surgical skills to deal with joint pathology. The second and third steps could be done using cadavers and/or virtual reality simulators (Fig. 10.2).

Bibliography

Alvand A, Auplish S, Gill H, Rees J (2011) Innate arthroscopic skills in medical students and variation in learning curves. J Bone Joint Surg Am 93(19):e115–e119, available from: PM:22005876

Andersen C, Winding TN, Vesterby MS (2011) Development of simulated arthroscopic skills. Acta Orthop 82(1):90–95, available from: PM:21281257

Bonrath EM, Fritz M, Mees ST, Weber BK, Grantcharov TP, Senninger N, Rijcken E (2013) Laparoscopic simulation training: does timing impact the quality of skills acquisition? Surg Endosc 27(3):888–894, available from: PM:23052509

Gallagher AG, Ritter EM, Champion H, Higgins G, Fried MP, Moses G, Smith CD, Satava RM (2005) Virtual reality simulation for the operating room: proficiency-based training as a paradigm shift in surgical skills training. Ann Surg 241(2):364–372, available from: PM:15650649

Harper JD, Kaiser S, Ebrahimi K, Lamberton GR, Hadley HR, Ruckle HC, Baldwin DD (2007) Prior video game exposure does not enhance robotic surgical performance. J Endourol 21(10):1207–1210, available from: PM:17949327

Howells NR, Gill HS, Carr AJ, Price AJ, Rees JL (2008) Transferring simulated arthroscopic skills to the operating theatre: a randomised blinded study. J Bone Joint Surg Br 90(4):494–499, available from: PM:18378926

Karam MD, Pedowitz RA, Natividad H, Murray J, Marsh JL (2013) Current and future use of surgical skills training laboratories in orthopaedic resident education: a national survey. J Bone Joint Surg Am 95(1):e4, available from: PM:23283381

Madan SS, Pai DR (2014) Role of simulation in arthroscopy training. Simul Healthc 9(2):127–135, available from: PM:24096921

Pedowitz RA, Esch J, Snyder S (2002) Evaluation of a virtual reality simulator for arthroscopy skills development. Arthroscopy 18(6):E29, available from: PM:12098111

Pernar LI, Smink DS, Hicks G, Peyre SE (2012) Residents can successfully teach basic surgical skills in the simulation center. J Surg Educ 69(5):617–622, available from: PM:22910159

Rosenthal R, Geuss S, Dell-Kuster S, Schafer J, Hahnloser D, Demartines N (2011) Video gaming in children improves performance on a virtual reality trainer but does not yet make a laparoscopic surgeon. Surg Innov 18(2):160–170, available from: PM:21245068

Snyder CW, Vandromme MJ, Tyra SL, Hawn MT (2009) Proficiency-based laparoscopic and endoscopic training with virtual reality simulators: a comparison of proctored and independent approaches. J Surg Educ 66(4):201–207, available from: PM:19896624

Strandbygaard J, Bjerrum F, Maagaard M, Winkel P, Larsen CR, Ringsted C, Gluud C, Grantcharov T, Ottesen B, Sorensen JL (2013) Instructor feedback versus no instructor feedback on performance in a laparoscopic virtual reality simulator: a randomized trial. Ann Surg 257(5):839–844, available from: PM:23295321

Thorson CM, Kelly JP, Forse RA, Turaga KK (2011) Can we continue to ignore gender differences in performance on simulation trainers? J Laparoendosc Adv Surg Tech A 21(4):329–333, available from: PM:21563940

Tuijthof GJ, van Sterkenburg MN, Sierevelt IN, Van OJ, van Dijk CN, Kerkhoffs GM (2010) First validation of the PASSPORT training environment for arthroscopic skills. Knee Surg Sports Traumatol Arthrosc 18(2):218–224, available from: PM:19629441

Wanzel KR, Ward M, Reznick RK (2002) Teaching the surgical craft: from selection to certification. Curr Probl Surg 39(6):573–659, available from: PM:12037512

Part III

Skills Performance Tracking

What Measures Represent Performance?

11

Tim Horeman, Kevin Sherman,
and Gabriëlle J.M. Tuijthof

Take Home Messages

- Motion- and time-based metrics can track instrument handling efficiency in endoscopy training.
- Force-based metrics can track tissue handling skills during training in endoscopy training.
- Motion, time and force information can be combined in specific metrics that indicate risks on hazards such as accidental tissue puncture or rupture.
- Metric-based post-task should be task dependent and easy to understand.
- Sufficient metrics are available to monitor training performance.

T. Horeman (✉)
Department of Biomechanical Engineering, Delft University of Technology, Delft, The Netherlands
e-mail: t.horeman@tudelft.nl

K. Sherman, MD
Department of Orthopedics, Castle Hill Hospital, Cottingham, East Yorkshire, UK
e-mail: kp_sherman@hotmail.com

G.J.M. Tuijthof
Department of Biomechanical Engineering, Delft University of Technology, Delft, The Netherlands

Department of Orthopedic Surgery, Academic Medical Centre, Amsterdam, The Netherlands
e-mail: g.j.m.tuijthof@tudelft.nl

11.1 Definitions

Assessing performance is one of the key elements that guide training and progress. To avoid discussions, the following definitions are made:

Metric, measure, parameter We define a metric as a quantity that in this context is supposed to reflect (part) of the performance of a trainee. Other terms that are considered as being synonym to a metric are *measure* and *parameter*.

Objective metrics are registered with sensors that are stand-alone or can be built-in a simulator. Optionally, the measured data from the sensors are post-processed to derive the metric.

Subjective metrics use expert judgments regarding performance behaviour. These can be partly objectified by scoring on rubrics using checklists.

Performance efficiency is an economic highly goal-oriented performance.

Performance safety is delicate tissue interaction and considerate instrument handling.

Proficiency in terms of instrument handling is defined as the optimal combination of performance efficiency and safety.

Direct feedback is given directly during the execution of a training task. Direct feedback is also named *real-time feedback*.

Post-task feedback is given after completion of a task. This type of feedback usually consists of several metrics and gives an overview of the entire task execution.

M. Karahan et al. (eds.), *Effective Training of Arthroscopic Skills*,
DOI 10.1007/978-3-662-44943-1_11, © ESSKA 2015

Subjective metrics are discussed in Chap. 13 as they are also suitable for application in the operating room to monitor complex tasks as they reflect a more holistic type of assessment.

11.2 Introduction

In previous chapters, the needs or training goals of arthroscopic skills were identified, as well as the possible means that is the various simulated training environments. This chapter focuses on the performance assessment or tracking of a trainee, which is the third key element required to provide a proper education environment. Establishing objective performance metrics is a challenging task, different approaches can be followed and many aspects influence the usability of a metric. One approach is to translate the training goals into measures; another approach is to translate psychomotor skills into measures. Both approaches require some form of decomposition into smaller elements that can be measured with a sensor. For example, the dexterity tools and tests described in Chap. 6 represent a decomposition into basic psychomotor skills that all can be measured with a single metric such as time. *However*, overall task performance of more complex tasks does not necessary equal the summation of the performance of several part-task goals or skills. Additionally, performance metrics should also be capable to discriminate between levels of expertise, easy to be interpreted, and to give directions to improve learning. One other aspect that should be taken into account is that objective metrics not only assess the performance of the trainees but also assess the performance of the simulator (Chap. 9). Bearing these considerations in mind, we do start by giving an overview of metrics that have been presented in literature to be useful in endoscopic training. They are categorized based on their suitability to represent performance efficiency or performance safety and suitability for direct or post-task feedback. Notice that not all presented metrics have been applied yet to training of arthroscopic skills. Based on this overview,

the translation is made towards performance tracking and feedback by discussing several examples.

A standard setting is introduced based upon which most metrics are presented graphically. Figure 11.1 shows an arthroscope and a probe that are inserted in a phantom knee joint. The path each tip of the instruments has moved for a period of 2.2 s is represented by the two 3D curves. The data are actual data from an evaluation test where a *navigate and probe task* was performed. The instruments are drawn in the mean direction of the travelled path. This example will be used throughout the section to illustrate the metrics concerning motion.

11.3 Metrics Reflecting Performance Efficiency

11.3.1 Task Repetition

The first quantitative metric is the number of task repetitions required to achieve a certain level of completion. This metric gives insight in the capability to learn in a new training environment and basically reflects the learning curve in time. Task repetition is one of the few metrics that does not require sensors to be objectively documented as long as the definition of *satisfactory completion* is clear. Therefore, the metric is highly suitable in different kinds of training programs (Scott et al. 2000).

11.3.2 Task Error

Similarly, to the number of task repetitions, the number of task errors can be documented without sensors. Examples of task errors can be the number of missed abnormalities or landmarks during an inspection task in the joint (Bliss et al. 2005; Hodgins and Veillette 2013; Sherman et al. 2001), the number of dropped objects from an instrument during a pick and remove task (Pellen et al. 2009; Rosser et al. 2006) or the number of misplaced suture insertions when performing

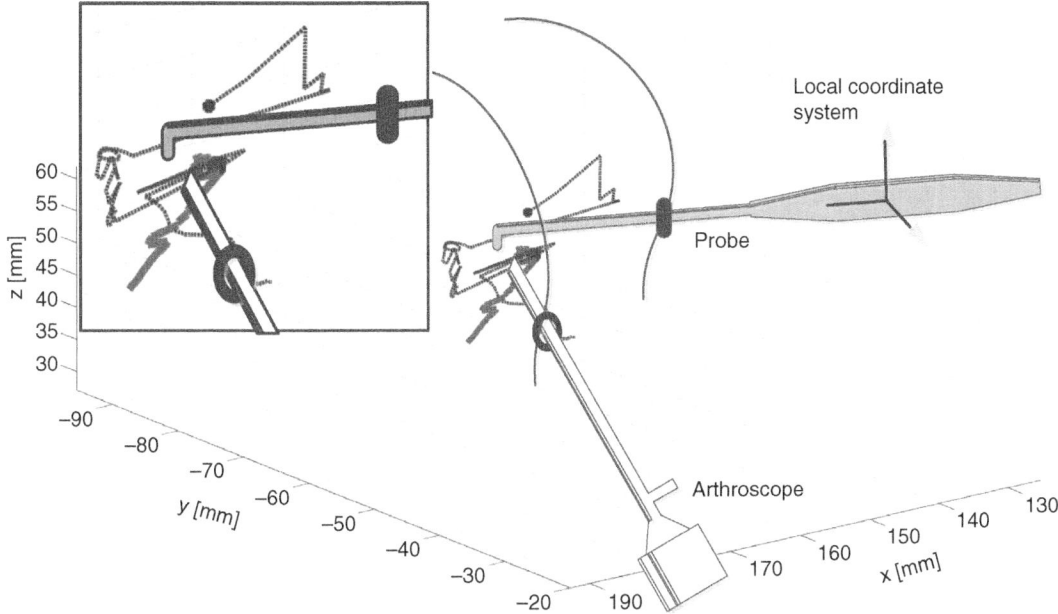

Fig. 11.1 Arthroscope and probe oriented in the lateral compartment of a phantom knee joint. The instruments are oriented in the mean direction of the travelled path.

The two 3D curves represent the travelled path for a period of 2.2 s of the arthroscope (*grey*) and probe (*black*), respectively. Start of the paths are marked

meniscal suturing. As is shown by the examples, the errors can be knowledge based or skill based and reflect performance in such a manner that it is also applicable in real-life surgery. Notice that the task errors should be well defined to be able to document their frequency.

11.3.3 Task Time

Task time (*t*) is defined as the period of time elapsed between the start of a task and the first second after completion of the task (Fig. 11.2):

$$t = t_{end} - t_{start}$$

Task time is found to be most discriminating between levels of experience as it highly reflects economy of motion (Andersen et al. 2011; Gomoll et al. 2008; Howells et al. 2008; Martin et al. 2011; Martin et al. 2012; McCarthy et al. 2006; Oropesa et al. 2013; Pedowitz et al. 2002; Tuijthof et al. 2010; Tuijthof et al. 2011b; Verdaasdonk et al. 2007). Advantages are that

task time is easy to understand and relatively easy to implement as it does not require high-end sensory equipment. A simple smartphone or timer is already sufficient.

11.3.4 Idle Time or State

Idle time (*it*) is defined as the percentage of the task time during which an instrument is held still (Chmarra et al. 2010; Oropesa et al. 2013). Idle state (*is*) is the number of instrument 'held stills' during task execution. For knee arthroscopy training, idle state was defined as the number of instances during which the subject looked away from the arthroscopy display unit to look at his or her hands while holding the arthroscope (Alvand et al. 2012).

Idle time or state reflects workflow interruptions due to a lack of knowledge (e.g. trainees hamper and do not know what kind of instrument to use) or task error (e.g. needle drops and need to be picked up). Therefore, this metric is in line with task time and path length in representing

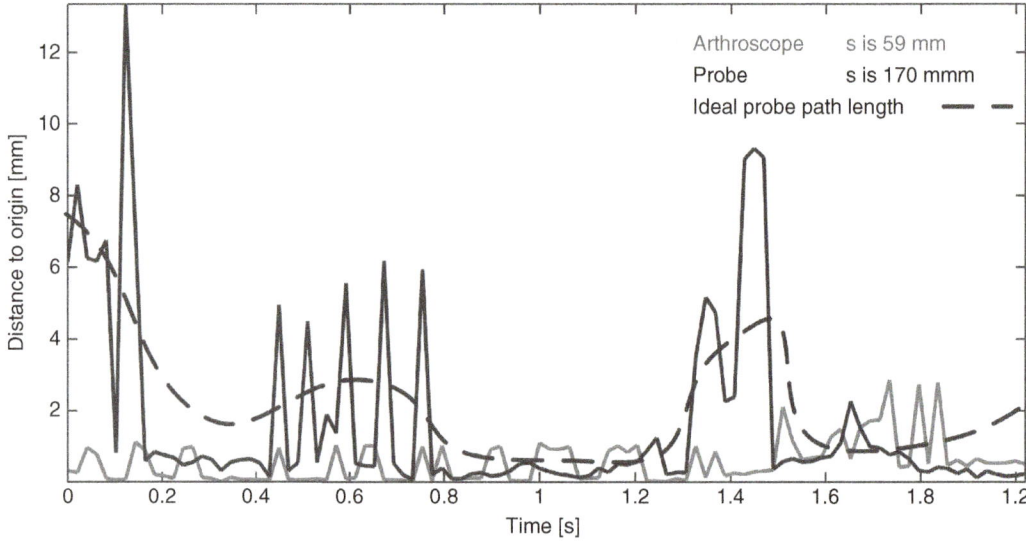

Fig. 11.2 Graphical presentation of task time, path length of arthroscope and probe and economy of movement, using the two 3D curves as presented in Fig. 11.1. The striped line shows an example of an ideal path length to demonstrate economy of movement

task efficiency. A study of Rosen and co-workers found that experts wasted less time between tissue manipulations in a box trainer compared with novices by looking at the idle states (Rosen et al. 1999).

11.3.5 Path Length

Path length (s) is defined as the total length of the path that the tip of an instrument or arthroscope has travelled in space (Fig. 11.2):

$$s = \sum_{i\,=\,start}^{end} \sqrt{\left(x_{i\,+\,1} - x_i\right)^2 + \left(y_{i\,+\,1} - y_i\right)^2 + \left(z_{i\,+\,1} - z_i\right)^2}$$

where the vectors x_i, y_i and z_i are the coordinates of the position in space of the tip for each time stamp. Physically, the path length can be measured by placing a rope at the start point and following the path with the rope until the end point. The total length of the rope needed to follow the trajectory is the path length of the instrument tip or arthroscope.

Path length is used as a measure to determine the efficiency of instrument and/or arthroscope motion (Andersen et al. 2011; Gomoll et al. 2007; Howells et al. 2008; McCarthy et al. 2006; Oropesa et al. 2013; Tashiro et al. 2009; Verdaasdonk et al. 2007). Path length has a role in goal orientation. Careful implementation of this parameter is required, as its value in reflecting performance depends on a well-defined trajectory. The reason is that experts do not necessarily take the shortest path to a target. This was nicely illustrated by Chmarra and co-workers (Chmarra et al. 2006). They found that a certain task had two clearly distinctive phases with the first being the 'seeking phase' when moving towards the target and the second being the 'retracting phase' when moving away from the target. Especially, in the 'seeking phase', differences were found between novices and experts with the experts demonstrating a significantly shorter path length, whereas the 'retracting phase' did not present differences.

Measuring the path length is easy when using virtual reality simulators as the simulated environment needs to know where the instrument is in the virtual space. So in order to let the simulation work, the orientation of the instruments is calculated anyhow and thus can be presented to the trainee. Tracking instrument motion in the physical world requires more effort, especially as a certain measurement accuracy is needed. Several tracking systems are indicated in Chap. 13, which can also be used in the operating room. A nice overview of tracking systems applied in endoscopic trainers is presented by Chmarra and co-workers (Chmarra et al. 2007). Once you have the 3D position data in time, other performance metrics can be deducted as well: economy of movement, motion volume, idle time, speed and smoothness.

11.3.6 Economy of Movement

Economy of movement (*em*) is defined as the percentage between the *ideal path length* (s_{ideal}) necessary to complete a task and the total path length (Bayona et al. 2008; Oropesa et al. 2013) (Fig. 11.2):

$$em = \frac{s_{ideal}}{s}$$

This implies that *em* gives a score between 0 and 100 %, with 100 % indicating *ideal economy of movement*. This metric is highly correlated to path length but compensates for the drawback of path length in defining the *ideal path length*, which is as indicated not necessarily the shortest length of the trajectory. Pedowitz and co-workers have used this metric and demonstrated differences between groups of different expertise (Pedowitz et al. 2002). A poor strategy to execute the task, task errors, steady hand, ambidexterity and manual precision are all technical skills that are reflected in the economy of motion metric.

11.3.7 Depth Perception

Depth perception (*dp*) is defined as the total distance travelled by an instrument along its longitudinal axis (Oropesa et al. 2013):

$$dp = \sum_{i = start}^{end} \sqrt{\left(l_{i+1} - l_i\right)^2}$$

With l_i being the distance for each time stamp. To determine *l*, the data first have to be oriented to the local coordinate system of the instrument, where one of the axes is defined in the direction of the longitudinal axis of the instrument (Fig. 11.1). Depth perception can be an indicator for poor instrument control when moving instruments perpendicular to the endoscopic image (Maithel et al. 2006; Rosen et al. 2006; Stylopoulos et al. 2004). This is caused by the fact that arthroscopic images are presented on a monitor showing a two-dimensional projection, whereas in reality instruments are navigated in a three-dimensional space inside the joint cavity. As this type of eye-hand coordination is completely different from everyday tasks, especially novices have difficulties in translating the three-dimensional environment to a two-dimensional representation, which results in poor positioning of the instrument tip. For application in arthroscopy, which uses a 30° angled arthroscope, *dp* should be determined of the instrument, and not of the arthroscope.

11.3.8 Volume of Motion

The volume of motion (V_{motion}) is defined as the volume of a 3D-dimensional ellipsoid spanned around the standard deviations of motion ($STD1_{motion}$, $STD2_{motion}$ and $STD3_{motion}$) along the three main directions of motion (Oropesa et al. 2013) (Fig. 11.3):

$$V_{motion} = \frac{4}{3}\pi\left(STD1_{motion} \bullet STD2_{motion} \bullet STD3_{motion}\right)$$

To determine the three main directions of motion, which do not necessarily coincides with the global coordinate system, a mathematical procedure is performed to convert the set of observations of possibly correlated variables into a set of values of uncorrelated variables called principal components (Chmarra et al. 2010; Horeman et al. 2012a). Subsequently, the standard deviations along those three main directions of motion are calculated and define the shape of the ellipsoid (Fig. 11.3).

Volume of motion is a measure for the space required by a trainee to complete the task. Similar as for path length, an *ideal volume of*

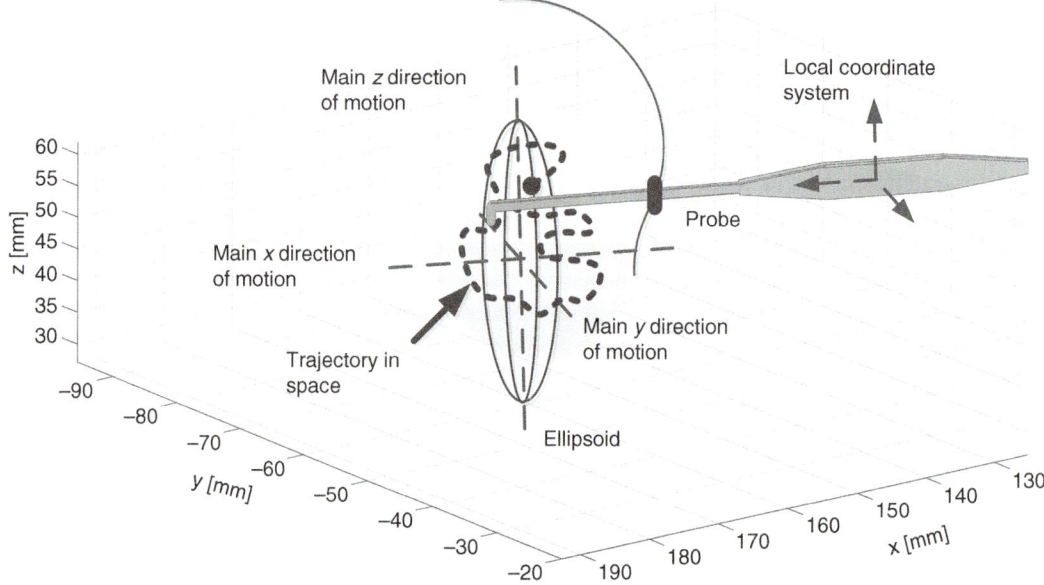

Fig. 11.3 Graphical presentation of the probe that is moved in 3D along a certain trajectory (*dotted line*). The solid lines represent a fitted ellipsoid which dimensions depend of motion (STD1 motion, STD2 motion and STD3 motion) along the three main directions of motion (indicated by straight dotted lines)

motion should be defined to compare trainee's performance with expert performance, as the smallest volume of motion does not necessarily reflect the optimal performance (Horeman et al. 2014b). Different from other metrics as path length, volume of motion is influenced by the direction of the instrument tip motion in three-dimensional space. For example, if the instrument tip is only moved along the instrument's longitudinal shaft, the path length increases, while the volume of motion remains zero until the instrument is also moved along all three axes of its local coordinate system.

11.4 Metrics Reflecting Performance Safety

11.4.1 Collision

A collision (*col*) is mostly defined as an instrument that unnecessarily touches surroundings. In this definition, a collision can be seen as a subset set of the metric task error, reflecting an error that potentially damages healthy tissue. So, the number of collisions reflects the number of times tissue might have been damaged during a task execution (Andersen et al. 2011; Gomoll et al. 2008; McCarthy et al. 2006; Pedowitz et al. 2002; Verdaasdonk et al. 2007). Similarly, to the path length, the number of collisions is a metric that is easily implemented in virtual reality simulators as this information needs to be determined to represent the virtual environment. Implementing collision detection in physical models is less straightforward. Some have applied electric wires that upon connection close an electric circuit which creates a buzz sound (Meyer et al. 1993; Tuijthof et al. 2003).

In other cases, collision detection can be determined based on the presence of certain force patterns in the recorded data (Horeman et al. 2014a). Collision detection can be based on the presence of frequencies in the recorded data for tasks such as pattern cutting, suturing and peg transfer in a box trainer (Smith et al. 1999). When applied for arthroscopy, such force frequency patterns might be detected when probing hard bony surfaces compared to probing softer fatty tissues, since the force build-up will be steeper in case of hard bone. It might be interesting to investigate if this theory can be applied, to distinguish between collision of instruments (hard surfaces) and collision with tissue (softer surfaces).

11.4.2 Out of View Time

The out-of-view time (*ovt*) is defined as the percentage of the task time that the instrument tip is not visible in the arthroscopic view (Horeman et al. 2014b), or as Alvand and co-workers defined "Prevalence of instrument loss" (Alvand et al. 2012). This metric reflects safety, as an instrument that is out of view can inflict unintended damage to the surrounding tissue when it is manoeuvred blindly. Out-of-view time can be quantified by analysis of recorded arthroscopic images. However, the out-of-view time can also be calculated if the 3D position and orientation

of the arthroscope and instrument are measured as can be done with 3D tracking systems. Also, the arthroscope's view angle and diameter need to be known. The latter two parameters define the view cone, which can be considered a volume in space (Fig. 11.4). Using the orientation of the arthroscope in space, the cone is attached in a fixed 30° angle to the tip of the arthroscope. Subsequently, it is verified if the coordinates of the instrument tip coincide with the cone for every time stamp by calculating the distance between the instrument tip and the outer surface of the view cone.

11.4.3 Tip-to-Tip Distance

The tip-to-tip distance (*t2td*) is defined as the distance between the arthroscope and the instrument tip for the entire task trajectory (Fig. 11.5):

$$t2td = \sum_{i\,=\,start}^{end} \sqrt{\left(x_{iscope} - x_{iprobe}\right)^2 + \left(y_{iscope} - y_{iprobe}\right)^2 + \left(z_{iscope} - z_{iprobe}\right)^2}$$

With x_i, y_i and z_i being the coordinates of the instruments' tips for every time stamp. This metric reflects the zone in which the manipulation takes place and is correlated with out-of-view time, since a high maximum tip-to-tip distance suggests that the instrument might be out of the

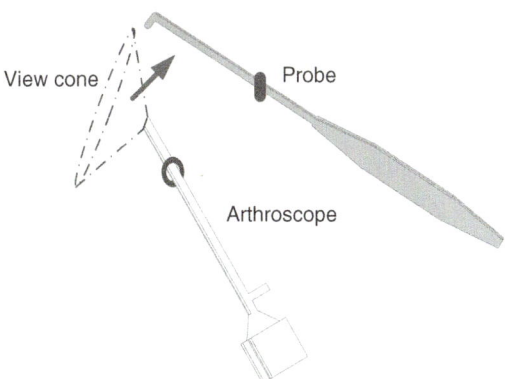

Fig. 11.4 Graphical presentation of the view cone of an arthroscope. The instrument has to be within this view cone to achieve full view time. The *arrow* indicates that the probe tip cannot be visualized by the arthroscope resulting in the start of registering the out-of-view time

arthroscopic view. This finding suggests that safe tissue handling is compromised.

Although the discriminating power of *t2td* depends highly on the type of task, a high mean tip-to-tip distance can inform the trainee to improve his/her overall safety performance during a task (Horeman et al. 2014b).

11.4.4 Motion Speed

In general, motion speed (*v*) is defined as the distance travelled per time (Oropesa et al. 2013) (Fig. 11.6):

$$v = \frac{s}{t}$$

where s is the path length and t is the time (e.g. task time).

Motion speed links position information to time information. In arthroscopy, the average motion speed has been used to assess performance (Gomoll et al. 2007, 2008), which reflects

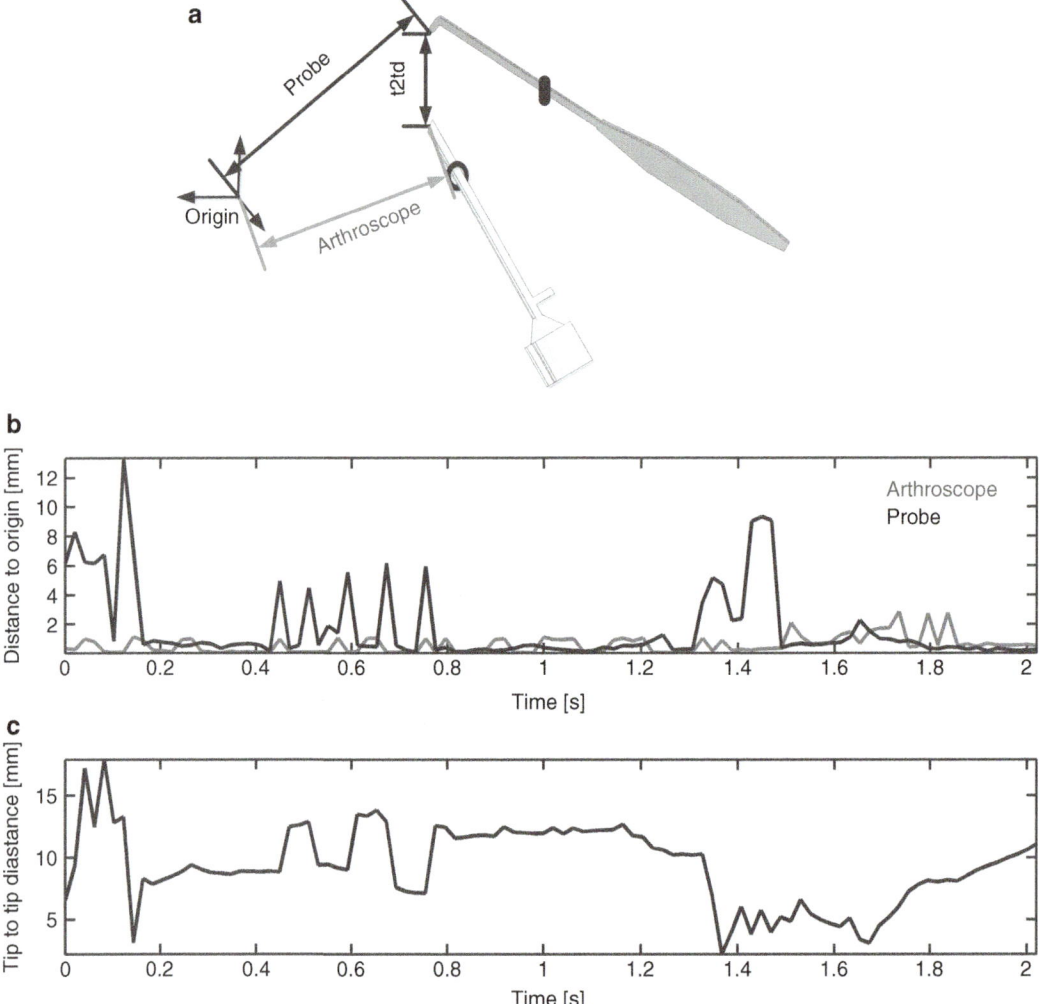

Fig. 11.5 (**a**) The tip-to-tip distance (*t2td*) is indicated in the sketch for one single time stamp. (**b**) The distance between point of origin and the distance to the instrument and arthroscope tips (Reproduced from Fig. 11.2). (**c**) From **b** the tip-to-tip distance curve is determined for this trajectory by subtraction of the distances between probe and arthroscope per time stamp

economy of movement. However, motion speed can also be used as follows. If the speed of the instruments is calculated per time stamp, the maximum speed can be determined for a training task. In a standard *position control* situation as is the case in robotic motion applications, a high instrument motion speed can be associated to overshoot and therefore poor position control. Returning to the clinical setting, instrument loading can build up due to contact between an instrument and the arthroscope or bony surface; when this loading is suddenly released, the instrument can overshoot and accidentally hit other tissues (Horeman et al. 2013). Thus, if uncontrolled instrument speeds occur during arthroscopy, it is possible that such events damage delicate anatomic structures around the operative zone. Due to force build-ups, instrument motion speed is linked to surgical safety (Horeman et al. 2013; Tarnay et al. 1999).

11.4.5 Motion Smoothness

Motion smoothness is defined as changes in instrument acceleration. Motion smoothness can

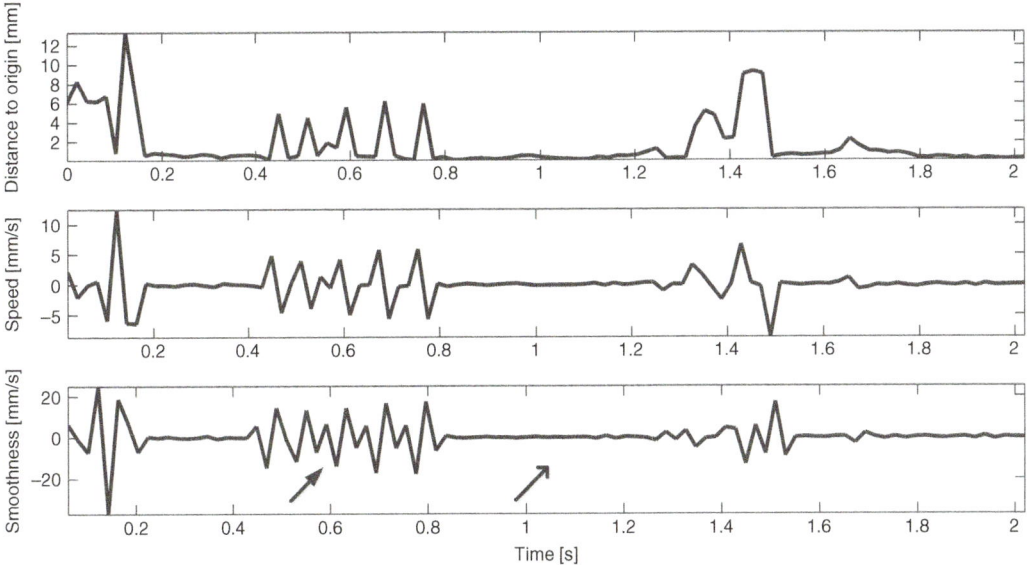

Fig. 11.6 Graphical presentation of the path length (s), the speed of motion (v) and motion smoothness (J) of the probe for the trajectory as presented in Fig. 11.1. In the motion smoothness curve, the closed arrow indicated a 'jerky' motion trajectory and the open arrow a *smooth* motion trajectory

be derived in various ways, we present one of the calculations suggested by Hogan and co-workers (Hogan and Sternad 2009), which is the root mean squared jerk (*J*) (Fig. 11.6):

$$ J = \sqrt{\frac{1}{t} \sum_{i\,=\,start}^{end} \left(\frac{\Delta^3 x_i}{\Delta t^3}\right)^2 + \left(\frac{\Delta^3 y_i}{\Delta t^3}\right) + \left(\frac{\Delta^3 z_i}{\Delta t^3}\right)} $$

with $\dfrac{\Delta^3 xi}{\Delta t^3}$, $\dfrac{\Delta^3 yi}{\Delta t^3}$ and $\dfrac{\Delta^3 zi}{\Delta t^3}$ being the third deriva-

tive of the x-, y- and z-position in time. A high motion smoothness suggests jerky movements of the surgical instrument (Oropesa et al. 2013), which again can compromise safe tissue manipulation.

11.4.6 Force Magnitude

Analogous to the indication of a position in space having an x, y and z component, the magnitude of a force is composed from its F_x, F_y and F_z magnitudes:

$$ F = \sqrt{\left(F_x + F_y + F_z\right)^2} $$

Besides quick and jerky motions, the force applied to surrounding tissue could lead to unintended damage of healthy tissue. This is especially true for healthy tissues in the intra-articular joint space that have limited healing potential (meniscus and cartilage) or vascular structures that heavily bleed. Tissue damage occurs if the tissue is loaded with magnitudes beyond the tissue's strength. Consequently, the force magnitude can qualify as a metric for monitoring safety. This suggests that calculation of the mean force exerted during a certain task might not sufficiently reflect safety performance. That is why the maximum peak force (Tashiro et al. 2009), as well as the standard deviation of forces (Chami et al. 2008; Horeman et al. 2010), and exceeding a certain threshold force (Obdeijn et al. 2014; Tuijthof et al. 2011a) have been suggested (Fig. 11.7). For all three options, significant differences were found between novices and experts.

The standard deviation of the (absolute) force indicates the ability of the trainee to apply a constant force on an object during a task. Especially in bimanual tasks as tissue stretching for dissection, anchor placement or needle driving a well-directed constant force on anchor, needle or tissue improves performance (Horeman et al. 2012a). Due to its nature, this component of the force is most informative in tasks that require

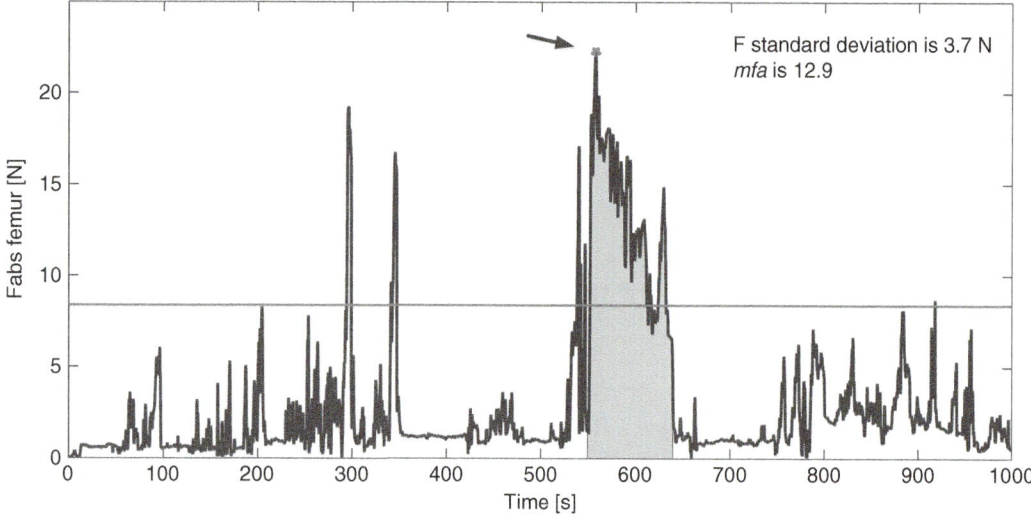

Fig. 11.7 Graphical presentation of the absolute force (F) when probing the femoral condyle in the PASSPORT simulator. Also the maximum peak force is indicated by the star (highlighted by the *arrow*), a threshold level is presented by the *grey line*, and the maximum force area (*mfa*) is indicated for this force pattern

continuous contact between instrument and task components.

Exceeding a certain threshold force is closely related to the collision metric but offers a more precise definition of the so-called collision as certain threshold needs to be exceeded for a certain period of time to qualify as collision (Fig. 11.7).

Measuring the actual forces during a task is not straightforward both in the virtual and the actual world. In virtual environments, haptic devices are used, which usually only give feedback on the tip forces. Also, their quality is not sufficient to mimic adequate haptic sensation, especially when machining of tissue is involved such as cutting, punching and drilling. In physical environments, instruments have been modified and equipped with sensors (Chami et al. 2006), 3D commercial force sensors that measure all force and moments (Tashiro et al. 2009) or a force platform that solely measure 3D reaction force of the tissue as result of instrument tissue manipulation (Horeman et al. 2010).

11.4.7 Force Direction

Analogous to the indication of a position in space having an x, y and z component, the direction of a force is composed from the ratios of the F_x, F_y and F_z magnitudes. An example is the expression of the force direction using two angles, with φ being defined as the direction of the force in the vertical plane:

$$tan\varphi = \frac{F_z}{F_y}$$

and γ being defined as the direction of the force in the horizontal plane.

$$tan\gamma = \frac{F_y}{F_x}$$

A study aimed to determine the force magnitude and directions exerted during arthroscopic navigation and inspection of a cadaver wrist showed that not so much the magnitude of the forces but the direction of the force differed significantly between experts and novices (Obdeijn et al. 2014). The experts executed forces containing a more perpendicular orientation on the cartilage tissue, whereas the novices executed forces containing a more shearing component. This might be an important difference, as navigation in the wrist is difficult due to the tide joint space and complex-shaped bones. In another study using the same setup of wrist arthroscopy training on a cadaveric specimen, it was found that novices did

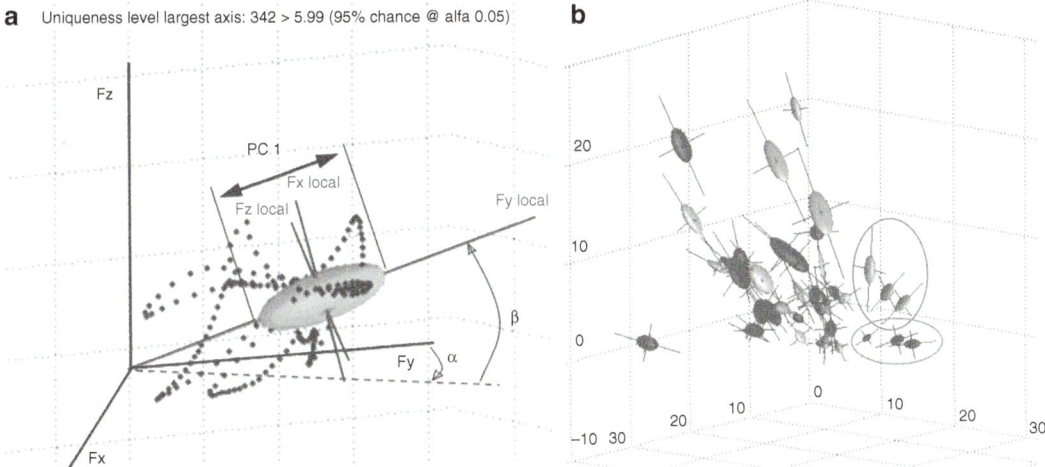

Fig 11.8 (**a**) 3D variability in forces. The *dots* represent the force in the global coordinate system (Fx, Fy, Fz). The ellipsoid is fitted on the force data and the orientation of PC1 force along Fx-local is defined by angles α and β. (**b**) Encircled ellipsoids of experts versus novices (not encircled) in a needle-driving task show that the force volume and direction can reveal consistency of an expert surgeon over three trials

not improve the loading of the tissues inside the wrist joint (Obdeijn et al. 2014). This suggests that force direction information can be indicative of a trainee's performance and the learning curve of novices.

11.4.8 Force Area

The maximum force area (*mfa*) is defined as the area of the absolute force peak in the force-time curve (Fig. 11.7):

$$mfa = \sum_{i=start}^{end} \sqrt{\left(F_{x,i} + F_{y,i} + F_{z,i}\right)^2}$$

With F_x, F_y and F_z being the x, y and z components of the force vector in space for every time stamp. In earlier work, *mfa* was referred to as force peak (Horeman et al. 2012a).

The starting time t_{start} and t_{end} can automatically be defined with different mathematical procedures, such as the point in time where the building of the absolute peak force is started or stopped, respectively, which can be deducted from the derivative of the force-time curve (Horeman et al. 2014b). The *mfa* indicates another aspect of the metric collision and can be considered as an elaboration of solely measuring

the peak force by taking into account its duration as well. Peak forces that are only applied for a brief time period (e.g. less than 0.5 s) might not inflict any damage, whereas a relative high force that is applied for a prolonged time period could cause tissue damage. As indicated before, the aptness of this measure compared to other safety-related performance measures depends on the task to be trained.

11.4.9 Volume of Force

The volume of force (V_{force}) is defined as the volume of a 3-dimensional ellipsoid spanned around the standard deviations of force ($STD1_{force}$, $STD2_{force}$, and $STD3_{force}$) along the three main directions of motion (Horeman et al. 2012a) (Fig. 11.8):

$$V_{force} = \frac{4}{3}\pi\left(STD1_{force} \cdot STD2_{force} \cdot STD3_{force}\right)$$

This definition as setup analogous to the metric 'volume of motion' as the same mathematical procedure (principal component analysis) can be applied to the x, y and z components of the force (Chmarra et al. 2010; Horeman et al. 2012a).

Volume of force is a measure for the forces required by a trainee to complete the task. Similar as for the volume of motion, an 'ideal volume of force' should be defined to compare trainee's performance with expert performance, as the smallest volume of motion does not necessarily reflect the optimal performance. The discriminative power of volume of force was determined in a study by Horeman and co-workers for an endoscopic suture task and confirmed (Horeman et al. 2012a).

11.5 Metrics Summary

Figure 11.9 shows how time, motion and force metrics inform about efficiency and safety performance. In endoscopic surgery, efficiency is reflected most strongly by task time, followed by the metrics task repetition and idle time. These three added with economy of movement indicate how fast the trainee adapts to a new situation when training. Another time-based parameter, out-of-view time, reflects safety performance. Distance metrics can inform both on efficiency performance (e.g. large or short path length to complete a task) and on safety performance (e.g. tip-to-tip distance). Force metrics measuring interaction forces during tissue manipulation can exclusively be associated to tissue damage

Table 11.1 Categorization of metrics

	Performance efficiency	Performance safety
Direct feedback	Task time	Collision
	Idle time	Tip-to-tip distance
	Path length	Motion speed
		Force magnitude
		Force direction
Post-task feedback	Task repetitions	Collision
	Task errors	Out-of-view time
	Task time	Tip-to-tip distance
	Idle time	Motion speed
	Path length	Smoothness
	Economy of movement	Force magnitude
	Volume of motion	Force direction
	Task errors	Force area
	Task time	Volume of force

(e.g. peak force, force threshold, force direction), but cannot inform on safe instrument handling if there is no interaction with the tissue. Since the above mentioned metrics are composed of single parameter measurement and need no post-calculation with mathematical procedures, they qualify to be used for direct feedback on performance (Table 11.1).

For other tasks, it can be helpful to use a metric that combines several parameters (Table 11.1). The combined information of time and motion is reflected by the metrics motion speed, motion smoothness and volume of motion. The combined information of time and force is reflected by the metrics force area and volume of force. These metrics of combined parameters tend to inform on safety performance (Table 11.1). The combined parameter metrics require post-processing or give a summary of the entire task performance, which makes them more suitable to use for post-task feedback.

11.6 Discussion

11.6.1 From Measuring Metrics to Training

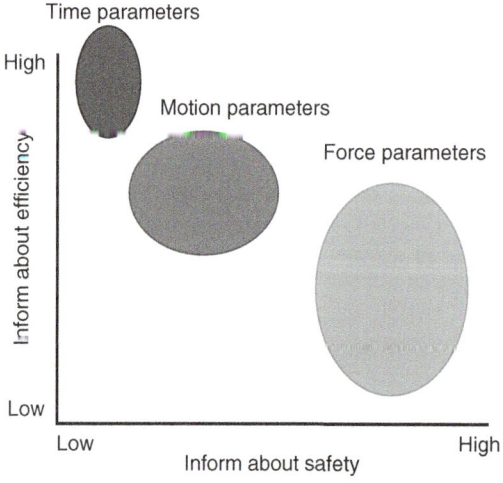

Direct feedback on performance is probably most relevant to apply in training, when on aims to learn A) how to follow a protocol or a certain

Fig. 11.9 The solid fields indicate the information that time and motion metrics can contain about efficiency and safety of a surgical action. The hatched field indicates the potential information that force metrics contain

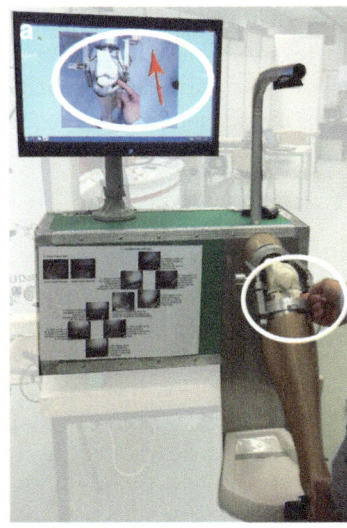
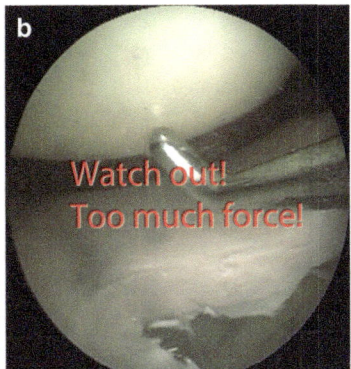
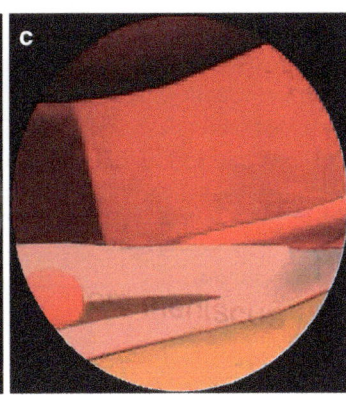

Fig. 11.10 (**a**) *Arrow* representation of the force magnitude and direction. The femoral condyle is pushed upward by the hand encircled in the right part of the picture; a resulting arrow is depicted on the interface screen to give visual feedback. (**b**) Textual guidance in PASSPORT user interface to guide a trainee to the next anatomic landmark. (**c**) Colouring red of the image in the SIMENDO arthroscopy, when tissue contact is too high. In all cases, the objects are displayed as an overlay on top of the arthroscopic image (© GJM Tuitjhof, 2014. Reprinted with permission)

sequence of manual actions and B) how to perform safe tissue manipulation (Table 11.1). For example, Horeman and co-workers have shown that novices can learn to endoscopically connect artificial tissue with less manipulation force by providing direct feedback of the force magnitude and direction (Horeman et al. 2012b).

When offering direct feedback, care has to be taken on how to inform the trainee and how to prevent mental overloading. The former depends on proper composition of the task and on defining the critical steps upon which should be reflected. Little to no literature on this aspect is available, other than general human factors and educational theories. For the latter, it should be noticed that people have three learning styles to receive and process information: oral, proprioceptive and visual (i.e. objects and text). Thus, all these type can be applied to give direct feedback. For oral feedback, an example was indicated for the collision metric where a buzz sound is given upon unallowed instrument tissue contact (Meyer et al. 1993; Tuijthof et al. 2003). Oral feedback in the form of alarms or buzzes is a common way to warn people that a dangerous situation is happening. This immediately poses a drawback to use in early learning stages of novices, as they are expected to make mistakes or errors at a frequent pace, which will set off the alarm signal many times during a task. If that happens, one tends to ignore such a signal and it no longer serves as adequate feedback signal. In multiple studies, researchers experimented to improve the sensation of the operating surgeons or to warn them if mistakes were made with haptic systems based on sensors, vibrating elements, motors and hydraulics (Westebring-van der Putten et al. 2008). For example, in the Daum-Hand (EndoHand) (Jackman et al. 1999; Melzer et al. 1997), the contact forces on the grasper were detected by membranes, amplified and transmitted hydraulically to membranes connected to the surgeon's fingertips to feel the average grasping force. A drawback of implementing such haptic way of giving feedback is that adding mass to the instrument handles or making modification to the instruments alters the instrument handling sensation which in itself is not ideal for training.

Visual or written feedback has also been implemented in arthroscopic simulators (Fig. 11.10). This is given in the form of object or text with or without colouring. In the study by Horeman and co-workers, the force direction and magnitude were simultaneously indicated by an arrow indicating the direction, its length, the size and its colour correct loading (Horeman et al. 2012b).

The real-time visual feedback in this study helps novices to choose the correct strategy on a skills- and knowledge-based level with information provided on a rule-based level (Dankelman et al. 2004; Wentink et al. 2003). This and other studies suggest that the human mind is capable of using additional visual information such as object colour and shape to improve tissue handling to some degree (Horeman et al. 2012b; Triano et al. 2006). Therefore, it seems that extra-visual information in the field of view of the trainee is easy to observe. On the other hand, if the visual feedback is given aside from the task area as presented on the screen, it can distract the trainee from the task or block other areas of interest. This aspect needs to be considered when simulating design, as during live surgery continuous focus is required on the surgical action. Thus, the manner in which feedback is given to the trainee is crucial to facilitate the training process.

So far, metrics have been presented that are more or less suitable for all or at least part of training tasks and can cover a wide range of different surgical actions. Concrete examples on how to use these for training arthroscopic skills are discussed.

The task time, tip-to-tip distance, motion smoothness and peak force can be applied in exercises where joint inspection is trained or tissue probing, and loose body removal. When punching or shaving meniscus tissue or executing meniscal suturing, the force area and volume of force can be applied, additionally. However, training of specific skills and tasks require additional performance assessment. For example, when performing a meniscectomy, it is highly relevant to measure the smoothness of the rim and the relative amount of removed tissue volume. This is possible but requires specific sensors (e.g. camera screenshots) and data processing. The last example is the training of drilling the holes in femur and tibia to prepare them for a cruciate ligament reconstruction. For this exercise, the direction of drilling is crucial. This could be measured by the direction of force, but in this case, the direction of the drill bit itself could indicate performance efficiency. This might be reflected by the sum of all angular rotation round the instrument's shaft length

(called angular path). Conclusively, the learning goals per task or exercise need to be clearly defined and the task needs to be clearly described, before choosing the proper metrics that reflect the performance.

11.6.2 Learning from Feedback

It is evident that not all metrics used for performance monitoring can be used for educational purposes. Trainees that receive feedback about their 'volume of force' or 'economy of motion' during a training session are not likely to transform this kind of information into better performance. Therefore, it is recommended to translate those metrics into constructive (task dependent) oral or written feedback to be understandable for the trainee. Table 11.2 shows how post-task feedback can be provided in between

Table 11.2 Metrics-based comprehensible feedback

Metric	Informative instruction to trainee
Task time	Task time is high; more practice is needed
Part length	Try to minimize unnecessary instrument movements
Speed	Slow your pace; decrease your instrument motion
Motion volume	Try to minimize unnecessary instrument movements
Tip-to-tip distance	Keep the instrument in sight. This avoids unintended damage to surrounding tissue
Out-of-view time	Keep the instrument in sight. This avoids unintended damage to surrounding tissue and speeds up your efficiency
Max force	Forces are too high. Minimize pushing or pulling during manipulation
	Avoid high insertion forces; your instrument is probably directed in a wrong manner
Mean force	Too much contact between instruments and tissue. Watch out for unintentional contact with tissue
Force Volume	Too much jerks or collisions during manipulation. Lower your instrument speed during manipulation
Max force area	Lower your force during insertion and tissue manipulation
	Keep your instrument tip in sight to avoid unintended tissue damage

trials. This schedule can truly lead to autonomous learning without the need to have a supervising surgeon standing next to the trainee.

Bibliography

Alvand A, Khan T, Al-Ali S, Jackson WF, Price AJ, Rees JL (2012) Simple visual parameters for objective assessment of arthroscopic skill. J Bone Joint Surg Am 94(13):e97, available from: PM:22760398

Andersen C, Winding TN, Vesterby MS (2011) Development of simulated arthroscopic skills. Acta Orthop 82(1):90–95, available from: PM:21281257

Bayona S, Fernandez-Arroyo JM, Martin I, Bayona P (2008) Assessment study of insight ARTHRO VR arthroscopy virtual training simulator: face, content, and construct validities. J Robot Surg 2(3):151–158

Bliss JP, Hanner-Bailey HS, Scerbo MW (2005) Determining the efficacy of an immersive trainer for arthroscopy skills. Stud Health Technol Inform 111:54–56, available from: PM:15718698

Chami G, Ward J, Wills D, Phillips R, Sherman K (2006) Smart tool for force measurements during knee arthroscopy: in vivo human study. Stud Health Technol Inform 119:85–89, available from: PM:16404020

Chami G, Ward JW, Phillips R, Sherman KP (2008) Haptic feedback can provide an objective assessment of arthroscopic skills. Clin Orthop Relat Res 466(4):963–968, available from: PM:18213507

Chmarra MK, Bakker NH, Grimbergen CA, Dankelman J (2006) TrEndo, a device for tracking minimally invasive surgical instruments in training setups. Sensors Actuators A Phys 126(2):328–334, available from: ISI:000235431800007

Chmarra MK, Grimbergen CA, Dankelman J (2007) Systems for tracking minimally invasive surgical instruments. Minim Invasive Ther Allied Technol 16(6):328–340, available from: PM:17943607

Chmarra MK, Klein S, de Winter JC, Jansen FW, Dankelman J (2010) Objective classification of residents based on their psychomotor laparoscopic skills. Surg Endosc 24(5):1031–1039, available from: PM:19915915

Dankelman J, Wentink M, Grimbergen CA, Stassen HG, Reekers J (2004) Does virtual reality training make sense in interventional radiology? Training skill-, rule- and knowledge-based behavior. Cardiovasc Intervent Radiol 27(5):417–421, available from: PM:15383842

Gomoll AH, O'Toole RV, Czarnecki J, Warner JJ (2007) Surgical experience correlates with performance on a virtual reality simulator for shoulder arthroscopy. Am J Sports Med 35(6):883–888, available from: PM:17261572

Gomoll AH, Pappas G, Forsythe B, Warner JJ (2008) Individual skill progression on a virtual reality simulator for shoulder arthroscopy: a 3-year follow-up study. Am J Sports Med 36(6):1139–1142, available from: PM:18326032

Hodgins JL, Veillette C (2013) Arthroscopic proficiency: methods in evaluating competency. BMC Med Educ 13:61, available from: PM:23631421

Hogan N, Sternad D (2009) Sensitivity of smoothness measures to movement duration, amplitude, and arrests. J Mot Behav 41(6):529–534, available from: PM:19892658

Horeman T, Rodrigues SP, Jansen FW, Dankelman J, van den Dobbelsteen JJ (2010) Force measurement platform for training and assessment of laparoscopic skills. Surg Endosc 24:3102–3108, available from: PM:20464416

Horeman T, Rodrigues SP, Jansen FW, Dankelman J, van den Dobbelsteen JJ (2012a) Force parameters for skills assessment in laparoscopy. IEEE Trans Haptics 5(4):312–322, available from: ISI:000310384300003

Horeman T, Rodrigues SP, van den Dobbelsteen JJ, Jansen FW, Dankelman J (2012b) Visual force feedback in laparoscopic training. Surg Endosc 26(1):242–248, available from: PM:21858573

Horeman T, Kurteva DDK, Valdastri P, Jansen FW, van den Dobbelsteen JJ, Dankelman J (2013) The influence of instrument configuration on tissue handling force in laparoscopy. Surg Innov 20(3):260–267, available from: PM:22956398

Horeman T, Blikkendaal MD, Feng D, Van DA, Jansen F, Dankelman J, van den Dobbelsteen JJ (2014a) Visual force feedback improves knot-tying security. J Surg Educ 71(1):133–141, available from: PM:24411436

Horeman T, Dankelman J, Jansen FW, van den Dobbelsteen JJ (2014b) Assessment of laparoscopic skills based on force and motion parameters. IEEE Trans Biomed Eng 61(3):805–813, available from: PM:24216633

Howells NR, Brinsden MD, Gill RS, Carr AJ, Rees JL (2008) Motion analysis: a validated method for showing skill levels in arthroscopy. Arthroscopy 24(3):335–342, available from: PM:18308187

Jackman SV, Jarzemski PA, Listopadzki SM, Lee BR, Stoianovici D, Demaree R, Jarrett TW, Kavoussi LR (1999) The EndoHand: comparison with standard laparoscopic instrumentation. J Laparoendosc Adv Surg Tech A 9(3):253–258, available from: PM:10414542

Maithel S, Sierra R, Korndorffer J, Neumann P, Dawson S, Callery M, Jones D, Scott D (2006) Construct and face validity of MIST-VR, Endotower, and CELTS: are we ready for skills assessment using simulators? Surg Endosc 20(1):104–112, available from: PM:16333535

Martin KD, Belmont PJ, Schoenfeld AJ, Todd M, Cameron KL, Owens BD (2011) Arthroscopic basic task performance in shoulder simulator model correlates with similar task performance in cadavers. J Bone Joint Surg Am 93(21):e1271–e1275, available from: PM:22048106

Martin KD, Cameron K, Belmont PJ, Schoenfeld A, Owens BD (2012) Shoulder arthroscopy simulator performance correlates with resident and shoulder arthroscopy experience. J Bone Joint Surg Am 94(21):e160, available from: PM:23138247

McCarthy AD, Moody L, Waterworth AR, Bickerstaff DR (2006) Passive haptics in a knee arthroscopy simulator: is it valid for core skills training? Clin Orthop Relat Res 442:13–20, available from: PM:16394733

Melzer A, Kipfmuller K, Halfar B (1997) Deflectable endoscopic instrument system DENIS. Surg Endosc 11(10):1045–1051, available from: PM:9381348

Meyer RD, Tamarapalli JR, Lemons JE (1993) Arthroscopy training using a "black box" technique. Arthroscopy 9(3):338–340, available from: PM:8323624

Obdeijn MC, Baalen SV, Horeman T, Liverneaux P, Tuijthof GJM (2014) The use of navigation forces for assessment of wrist arthroscopy skills level. J Wrist Surg 3:132–138

Oropesa I, Chmarra MK, Sanchez-Gonzalez P, Lamata P, Rodrigues SP, Enciso S, Sanchez-Margallo FM, Jansen FW, Dankelman J, Gomez EJ (2013) Relevance of motion-related assessment metrics in laparoscopic surgery. Surg Innov 20(3):299–312, available from: PM:22983805

Pedowitz RA, Esch J, Snyder S (2002) Evaluation of a virtual reality simulator for arthroscopy skills development. Arthroscopy 18(6):E29, available from: PM:12098111

Pellen MG, Horgan LF, Barton JR, Attwood SE (2009) Construct validity of the ProMIS laparoscopic simulator. Surg Endosc 23(1):130–139, available from: PM:18648875

Rosen J, MacFarlane M, Richards C, Hannaford B, Sinanan M (1999) Surgeon-tool force/torque signatures – evaluation of surgical skills in minimally invasive surgery. Stud Health Technol Inform 62:290–296, available from: PM:10538374

Rosen J, Brown JD, Chang L, Sinanan MN, Hannaford B (2006) Generalized approach for modeling minimally invasive surgery as a stochastic process using a discrete Markov model. IEEE Trans Biomed Eng 53(3):399–413, available from: PM:16532766

Rosser JC Jr, Colsant BJ, Lynch PJ, Herman B, Klonsky J, Young SM (2006) The use of a "hybrid" trainer in an established laparoscopic skills program. JSLS 10(1):4–10, available from: PM:16709348

Scott DJ, Bergen PC, Rege RV, Laycock R, Tesfay ST, Valentine RJ, Euhus DM, Jeyarajah DR, Thompson WM, Jones DB (2000) Laparoscopic training on bench models: better and more cost effective than operating room experience? J Am Coll Surg 191(3):272–283, available from: PM:10989902

Sherman KP, Ward JW, Wills DP, Sherman VJ, Mohsen AM (2001) Surgical trainee assessment using a VE knee arthroscopy training system (VE-KATS): experimental results. Stud Health Technol Inform 81:465–470, available from: PM:11317792

Smith S, Wan A, Taffinder N, Read S, Emery R, Darzi A (1999) Early experience and validation work with

Procedicus VA – the Prosolvia virtual reality shoulder arthroscopy trainer. Stud Health Technol Inform 62:337–343, available from: PM:10538383

Stylopoulos N, Cotin S, Maithel SK, Ottensmeye M, Jackson PG, Bardsley RS, Neumann PF, Rattner DW, Dawson SL (2004) Computer-enhanced laparoscopic training system (CELTS): bridging the gap. Surg Endosc 18(5):782–789, available from: PM:15216861

Tarnay CM, Glass KB, Munro MG (1999) Entry force and intra-abdominal pressure associated with six laparoscopic trocar-cannula systems: a randomized comparison. Obstet Gynecol 94(1):83–88, available from: PM:10389723

Tashiro Y, Miura H, Nakanishi Y, Okazaki K, Iwamoto Y (2009) Evaluation of skills in arthroscopic training based on trajectory and force data. Clin Orthop Relat Res 467(2):546–552, available from: PM:18791774

Triano JJ, Scaringe J, Bougie J, Rogers C (2006) Effects of visual feedback on manipulation performance and patient ratings. J Manipulative Physiol Ther 29(5):378–385, available from: PM:16762666

Tuijthof GJM, van Engelen SJMP, Herder JL, Goossens RHM, Snijders CJ, van Dijk CN (2003) Ergonomic handle for an arthroscopic cutter. Minim Invasive Ther Allied Technol 12(1–2):82–90, available from: ISI:000184323300012

Tuijthof GJ, van Sterkenburg MN, Sierevelt IN, Van OJ, van Dijk CN, Kerkhoffs GM (2010) First validation of the PASSPORT training environment for arthroscopic skills. Knee Surg Sports Traumatol Arthrosc 18(2):218–224, available from: PM:19629441

Tuijthof GJ, Horeman T, Schafroth MU, Blankevoort L, Kerkhoffs GM (2011a) Probing forces of menisci: what levels are safe for arthroscopic surgery. Knee Surg Sports Traumatol Arthrosc 19(2):248–254, available from: PM:20814661

Tuijthof GJ, Visser P, Sierevelt IN, van Dijk CN, Kerkhoffs GM (2011b) Does perception of usefulness of arthroscopic simulators differ with levels of experience? Clin Orthop Relat Res, available from: PM:21290203

Verdaasdonk EG, Stassen LP, Schijven MP, Dankelman J (2007) Construct validity and assessment of the learning curve for the SIMENDO endoscopic simulator. Surg Endosc 21(8):1406–1412, available from: PM:17653815

Wentink M, Stassen LP, Alwayn I, Hosman RJ, Stassen HG (2003) Rasmussen's model of human behavior in laparoscopy training. Surg Endosc 17(8):1241–1246, available from: PM:12799883

Westebring-van der Putten EP, Goossens RH, Jakimowicz JJ, Dankelman J (2008) Haptics in minimally invasive surgery – a review. Minim Invasive Ther Allied Technol 17(1):3–16, available from: PM:18270873

What Thresholds Are Evidence Based?

12

Gabriëlle J.M. Tuijthof and Tim Horeman

Take-Home Messages

- Thresholds for time-, motion- and force-based metrics are required to facilitate training and to set uniform standards for assessment.
- Thresholds can be derived from theoretic calculations, tissue experiments or from measurements with experts.
- Specific research is required to determine evidence-based sets of thresholds that can be used for training.

12.1 Definitions

As discussed in Chap. 11, assessing performance is key to guide and monitor training and progression. Apart from measuring objective metrics, thresholds need to be determined that represent proficiency. To avoid discussions, the following definitions are made:

Task or exercise is a combined set of necessary (arthroscopic) actions to achieve the goal as requested by the task.

G.J.M. Tuijthof (✉)
Department of Biomechanical Engineering, Delft University of Technology, Delft, The Netherlands

Department of Orthopedic Surgery, Academic Medical Centre, Amsterdam, The Netherlands
e-mail: g.j.m.tuijthof@tudelft.nl

T. Horeman
Department of Biomechanical Engineering, Delft University of Technology, Delft, The Netherlands
e-mail: t.horeman@tudelft.nl

Proficiency in terms of instrument handling is defined as the optimal combination of performance efficiency and safety (Chap. 11).

Threshold is the magnitude or intensity that must be exceeded for a certain condition to occur or be manifested; but a thresholds means also the maximum level of magnitude considered to be acceptable or safe (Oxford English Dictionary 2014).

Tissue damage is defined as macroscopically visible tearing or rupturing of tissue.

12.2 Introduction

In this section of the book, we still focus on simulator training, that is, training outside the operating room on any type of simulated environment using any of the presented metrics. This chapter is a directly related to Chap. 11, since performance tracking is less useful if no clear indications can be given to the trainees if and when they have achieved proficiency to continue the next phase of training. To feed this information back to the trainee without frequent supervision of teaching staff, thresholds need to be set for the objective performance metrics. With this, we leave the domain of simulator validation and enter the domain of task design and validation. Similar to determining metrics that best reflect a certain task performance, determining complementary thresholds is a tedious task for several reasons. First, tasks need to be precisely defined by decomposing them in smaller elements, whereas in actual performance of arthroscopy several approaches can usually be applied without affecting the surgical outcome. An example is the presence of various techniques to execute meniscus suturing (Cho 2014; Forkel et al. 2014; Ra et al. 2013) or approaches to access the shoulder joint (Meyer et al. 2007; Soubeyrand et al. 2008). Second, some thresholds, such as task time, depend on the task, which requires them to be determined per task. This was, for example, done by Schreuder and co-workers who evaluated all five exercises available on a VR simulator for training of laparoscopic skills (Schreuder et al. 2011) with complementary metrics for each specific exercise. Third, sometimes it is difficult to determine the optimal performance efficiency, which is required to set thresholds. Finally, when using thresholds for direct feedback settings, care has to be taken how to inform the trainee and how to prevent mental overloading.

Nevertheless, determination of evidence-based thresholds highly supports the availability of validated simulator training curricula that offer exercises that truly discriminate between levels of experience. Eventually, this supports uniformity in performance tracking and objective definition of levels of proficiency. This could lead to summative testing of innate arthroscopic skills of future residents before being accepted into a residency programme (Alvand et al. 2011) and of basic arthroscopic skills to qualify for continued training in the operating room. Two methods are presented to determine thresholds for different types of metrics and illustrated with examples.

12.3 Theoretic Thresholds

The term *theoretic* indicates the possibility to calculate the *ideal* or at least the *extreme* magnitude or setting of a metric for a given task. This method is widely applied in robotic control, for example, when a robot arm needs to move via the shortest trajectory from location A to location B or within the fastest possible time. The terms *shortest* and *fastest* indicate the extreme of the magnitude calculated with the shortest trajectory from location

A to location B, the dimensions and degrees of freedom of the robotic arm as well as positions in space of the locations of A and B are assumed to be known. In the remainder of this section, several examples are given of theoretic thresholds that can be derived both for performance efficiency and performance safety metrics. This illustrates how this approach can be applied for training of arthroscopic skills.

12.4 Idle Time, Out of View Time and Motion Smoothness

Idle time can be used as metric if a threshold is set that defines 'still'. Its theoretic threshold is easily derived by demanding that the instrument tip never remains in one freeze position during task execution or demanding that the instrument tip motion speed never is zero for a certain time. Similarly, the theoretic threshold for out of view time can be derived to be zero as well. This implies that the position of the instrument remains always in the view cone of the arthroscope (Fig. 11.4). Finally, another easy to derive theoretic threshold is that of motion smoothness which is zero, as this requires the instrument to show no changes in its motion acceleration. The theoretic determined thresholds for these three metrics are determined independently of a certain task.

12.5 Path Length

To demonstrate how the metric path length can be determined, we use a simplified navigation task in this example. Suppose that for this navigation task, it is required to navigate and probe five anatomic landmarks: medial tibia plateau (1), posterior horn of the medical meniscus (2), midsection of the anterior cruciate ligament (3), lateral tibia plateau (4) and posterior horn of the lateral meniscus (5) (Fig. 12.1). We assume that these five landmarks are located in a single plane. Subsequently, the shortest total path length (*smin*) to probe all landmarks in the predefined sequence can be calculated:

$$s\,\mathrm{min} = \sum_{i=1}^{s} \sqrt{\left(x_{i+1} - x_i\right)^2 + \left(y_{i+1} - y_i\right)^2}$$

where the x_i and y_i are the coordinates of each of the five landmark positions in the plane. *Smin* is the absolute minimal path length for the given trajectory. This means that there is no other option to following this trajectory in an even shorter manner. So, trainees can be requested to exactly follow this trajectory with the tip of their instrument to execute this particular task. This example illustrates the task dependence of the set threshold, since another navigation task can give another magnitude of *smin*.

12.6   Force Magnitude

Safe tissue manipulation was associated with force magnitudes used to load tissues (Chap 9). It was stated that tissue damage occurs if the tissue is loaded beyond the tissue's material strength. Material strength is a tissue material property that indicates the failure level. This failure property will be used to determine theoretic thresholds for two types of tissues: meniscal and ligamentous tissue. Setting a threshold for safe meniscus probing is relevant to stimulate safe manipulation of this delicate tissue, since it has little to no healing potential (Tuijthof et al. 2011). Setting a threshold for safe ligament loading is relevant for arthroscopic training; the lower leg is stressed during knee arthroscopies to increase the available joint space. Ligament failure can be prevented if maximum loading levels are not exceeded (Stunt et al. 2013). Calculation of the force magnitude is only possible if tissue material properties, volume and their contact areas with instruments are known. If not, tissue properties should first be determined from experiments (e.g. (Tuijthof et al. 2009)). Additionally, tissue measurements and observation studies are required to determine the manipulated tissue's cross-sectional area's and contact surfaces.

All tissues, thus meniscal and ligamentous tissue as well, present a viscoelastic behaviour with a nonlinear relation between force and displacement (Buchner 2009; Chmarra et al. 2006;

Fithian et al. 1990; Hull et al. 1996; Kennedy et al. 1976; Robinson et al. 2005). When loading the tissue, the tissue starts to deform elastically, followed by plastic deformation. Finally, when the load exceeds, the material's failure property either pure shearing or tearing causes tissue to rupture (Tuijthof et al. 2011). To set the theoretic thresholds, the variation in tissue material properties amongst the human population needs to be taken into account. The aim is to set force magnitude thresholds that prevent damaging even the weakest tissue when performing tissue manipulation. Consequently, the failure property of these weakest tissues should be determined, which is derived by subtracting three times the standard deviation from the mean failure property (Tuijthof et al. 2009). This should cover 99 % of the normal human population. Subsequently, the minimum force is determined to actually rupture the weakest tissues using values from tensions studies performed with human cadaver material (Kennedy et al. 1976; Robinson et al. 2005; Trent et al. 1976; Tuijthof et al. 2009). A threshold value of 8.5 N has been derived for probing of meniscus tissue (illustrated in Fig. 11.7) (Tuijthof et al. 2011), and a threshold value of 78 N has been derived for stressing the lower leg at the level of the ankle

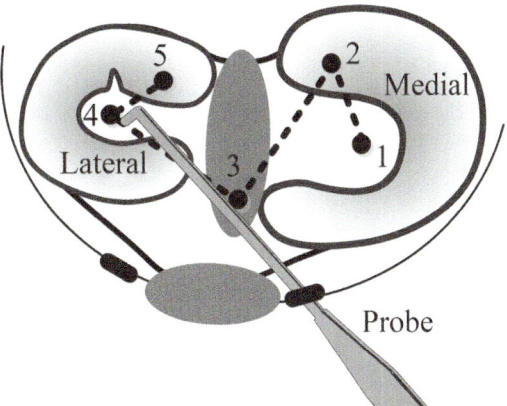

Fig. 12.1 Cross-sectional view of a knee joint showing the lateral and medial menisci, the anterior cruciate ligament zone (*grey* area) and the portals. The numbered bullets indicate the five landmarks that need to be probe for the set navigation task in the indicated sequence. The *dotted line* represents *smin*, which is the minimal path length of the trajectory to probe the landmarks

joint (Stunt et al. 2013). Thus, remaining below these theoretic threshold levels minimises the chance to damage tissue unintentionally.

12.7   Expert Thresholds

Another approach to set thresholds for performance metrics is using values acquired from experts performing tasks in the simulated environment. The line of reasoning supporting this approach is that experts have reached the plateau in their learning curve and demonstrate proficiency in arthroscopic skills. Thus, their task performance reflects the optimal manner to execute that particular task. To document reliable data, experts should have gotten the opportunity to familiarise themselves with the simulated environment and the task, and their number should be sufficiently large to minimise the influence of outliers.

Even with these preconditions taken into account, there is room for subjective selection of the threshold levels, e.g. the mean value, the mean added or subtracted with n times the standard deviation, the median, minimum or maximum values of the expert data sets. In the remainder of this section, several examples are given of expert thresholds that can be derived both for performance efficiency and performance

safety metrics. This illustrates how this approach can be applied for training of arthroscopic skills.

12.8   Performance Efficiency Metrics

Task time (t), path length (s) and economy of motion (em) were the performance efficiency metrics for which we found expert data sets (Tables 12.1 and 12.2). These expert data sets were not the goal of these studies but were acquired to assess construct validity of arthroscopic knee and shoulder simulators. Nevertheless, these are the only sets from which quantitative thresholds can be derived.

The process how the expert data were utilised to form both tables is elucidated. Only tasks were included that were explicitly described. If possible, only the last trial in a series of repetitive trials was processed, to minimise possible bias due to familiarisation. Only expert data were included that gave significantly different results compared to less experienced groups. If the same tasks were performed on different simulators or investigated in multiple studies, the results were pooled as follows. The mean values of each metric were calculated by the weighted mean using the relative number of experts per study as weighing factor.

Table 12.1 Experts threshold levels determined for tasks and performance efficiency metrics of knee simulators

Task	Simulator(s)	Expert characteristics	Metrics	Threshold μ	Threshold μ-σ
Find five loose bodies (McCarthy et al. 2006)	SKATS knee	n=12	t	243 s.	124 s.
		Faculty fellows	sscope	168 cm	70 cm
		>1,000 arthroscopies	sprobe	156 cm	74 cm
Navigate and probe nine landmarks (Fig. 7.3) (Tuijthof et al. 2010)	ArthoSim™, Arthro Mentor™, PASSPORT, VirtaMed ArthroS™ (Ch. 7), all knees	n=31 >60 arthroscopies Only last trial	t	36 s.	21 s.
Navigate and probe 10 landmarks (Tashiro et al. 2009)	Sawbones™ knee	n=6 faculty	t	199 s.	144 s.
			sscope	382 cm	293 cm
			sprobe	49 cm	36 cm
Partial meniscectomy (Tashiro et al. 2009)	Sawbones™ knee	n=6 faculty	t	299 s.	223 s.
			sscope	489 cm	318 cm
			spunch	966 cm	789 cm
Diagnostic arthroscopy (Cannon et al. 2014)	ArthoStim™	n=6 faculty	t	610 s.	

The metrics are indicated by the symbols used in Chap. 9. For each data set, options for threshold setting are indicated. μ is mean value, σ is standard deviation

Table 12.2 Experts threshold levels determined for tasks and performance efficiency metrics of shoulder simulators

Task	Simulator	Expert characteristics	Metrics	Threshold μ	Threshold CI
Navigate and probe 11 landmarks (Gomoll et al. 2007; Pedowitz et al. 2002)	Procedicus™ shoulder	$n = 31$ Faculty fellows	t em	52 s. 268 %	μ-σ = 30 s μ-σ = 189 %
Navigate and probe nine landmarks (Howells et al. 2008)	Sawbones™ shoulder	$n = 5$ >101 arthroscopies	t sscope + sprobe	46 s. 85 cm	26 s. 55 cm
Grasp and remove a 3 mm ball (Howells et al. 2008)	Sawbones™ shoulder	$n = 5$ >101 arthroscopies	t sscope + sprobe	24 s. 77 cm	13 s. 59 cm
Navigate and probe landmarks 'Blue sphere' (Andersen et al. 2011)	Arthro Mentor™ shoulder	$n = 7$ >1 arthroscopy independently per week Only last trial	t sscope sprobe	223 s. 84 cm 103 cm	118 s. 43 cm 42 cm

The metrics are indicated by the symbols used in Chap. 9. For each data set, options for threshold setting are indicated. μ is mean value, σ is standard deviation, CI is lowest level of 95 % confidence interval

These mean values (μ) are presented as a first possible threshold (Tables 12.1 and 12.2 all but last column). Subsequently, the largest standard deviation (or lowest 95 % confidence level) of each metric was selected to define a second possible threshold: mean value subtracted by the standard deviation (μ-σ) (Tables 12.1 and 12.2 last column). Subtraction of the standard deviation was used, this results in lower threshold values, which implies that trainees need to demonstrate increased performance efficiency.

When analysing the tables, the following remarks can be made:

> The number of experts is limited and inconsistently defined in the studies.
> The number of tasks is limited to predominantly navigation and probe tasks.
> The order of magnitude of the task times and path lengths is quite similar for the navigation tasks, which implies a certain level of consistency.

12.9 Performance Safety Metrics

12.9.1 Experimentally Defined Thresholds

As alternative for calculating the force magnitude based on known tissue properties as described in the previous paragraph, force parameters that represent tissue damage can also be determined based on tissue measurements. This is especially useful when there are too many unclear factors that prevent reliable calculation of the force magnitude threshold. Especially when the conditions during loading are relatively constant (e.g. knowing the grasping surface of a grasper or the contact area between needle and tissue during suturing), it is possible to mimic the surgical action for multiple tissue samples in a test setup to measure the maximal loading force before tissue rupture(Heijnsdijk et al. 2004; Rodrigues et al. 2012). By taking enough tissue samples from multiple individuals, the combined factors of influence are considered as 'black box', while statistics are used on the measurement outcomes to find the maximal allowable force for force critical surgical action as drilling, suturing or tissue handling. According to the known literature, this approach was not used yet to determine the maximal allowable force magnitude for arthroscopic tissue structures.

12.9.2 Thresholds Derived from Literature

Following the same process as executed to form the tables of the performance efficiency thresholds, a table with performance safety thresholds

Table 12.3 Experts threshold levels determined for tasks and performance safety metrics of knee simulators

Task	Simulator	Expert characteristics	Metrics	Threshold μ	Threshold μ+σ
Navigate and probe landmarks *blue sphere* (Andersen et al. 2011)	Arthro Mentor™ shoulder	$n=7$ >1 arthroscopy independently per week Only last trial	col	68	CI=106
Navigate and probe 10 landmarks (Tashiro et al. 2009)	Sawbones™ knee	$n=6$ faculty	vscope	2.2 cm/s	2.7 cm/s
			vprobe	2.7 cm/s	3.1 cm/s
			Fmax	11.7 N	16 N
			Fmean	2.4 N	2.9 N
			mfa	455 Ns	594 Ns
Partial meniscectomy (Tashiro et al. 2009)	Sawbones™ knee	$n=6$ faculty	vscope	1.7 cm/s	2.1 cm/s
			vprobe	3.3 cm/s	3.9 cm/s
			Fmax	22.7 N	28.7 N
			Fmean	4.4 N	5.4 N
			mfa	1372 Ns	1943 Ns
Meniscus push (Tuijthof et al. 2011)	Cadaver tissue	$n=3$ >250 arthroscopies per year	Fmax	3.2 N	4.1 N
Meniscus sweep (Tuijthof et al. 2011)	Cadaver tissue	$n=3$ >250 arthroscopies per year	Fmax	2.8 N	3.1 N
Meniscus pull (Tuijthof et al. 2011)	Cadaver tissue	$n=3$ >250 arthroscopies per year	Fmax	4.1 N	5.2 N
Joint stressing (Stunt et al. 2013)	In vivo 21 patients	$n=2$ >250 arthroscopies per year	Fmax	60 N	88 N

The metrics are indicated by the symbols used in Chap. 11. For each data set, options for threshold setting are indicated. μ is mean value, σ is standard deviation, CI is 95 % confidence interval

was made including the metrics: collisions (*col*), motion speed (*v*), force magnitude (*F*) and force area (*mfa*) (Table 12.3). Two aspects are different compared to Tables 10.1 and 10.2, which are elucidated.

First, the last column contains values where the standard deviation was added to the mean value to a second threshold. This results in threshold values that seem to be less strict in terms of defining safe tissue manipulation. However, as the values are from experts, we can argue that these levels should be safe. Second, two studies were performed with the goal to determine safe manipulation thresholds for meniscal and ligamentous tissue, which was determined in vitro and in vivo (Stunt et al. 2013; Tuijthof et al. 2011). When analysing Table 12.3, the same remarks can be made as presented for the performance efficiency metrics, except that the suggested levels for tissue probing and joint stressing are based on a higher level of evidence.

12.10 Discussion

Two methods were presented to derived evidence-based thresholds for training of tasks in simulated environments: the theoretic and experimental expert approach. Examples were given how to determine theoretic thresholds for both efficiency and safety metrics, for which the latter requires knowledge on material properties of human tissue. Data of experts from which thresholds could be derived is marginally available in literature (Tables 12.1, 12.2 and 12.3). Both methods have pros and cons, with theoretic thresholds being too strict at times and expert-derived thresholds requiring still a subjective decision which level to use. Therefore, it is suggested to combine both methods to set realistic and evidence-based thresholds. Two examples are given.

The application of the theoretic threshold for path length (*smin*) might be too strict, since no deviation from *smin* is allowed, which is almost impossible to achieve. This could evoke unrealistic or undesired performance behaviour to achieve task completion, such as extreme slow movement of the probe. Also, it could cause frustration as trainees find it impossible to achieve the required threshold and might get demotivated to continue training. So, rather than using such 'extreme' theoretic threshold, its magnitude can be used as a starting value to set a threshold which is defined by faculty or can be used to decide which expert values (mean, mean added or subtracted with standard deviation) too be used. Additionally, if expert and theoretic threshold values deviate too much, further analysis could highlight performance strategies which not necessarily strive to minimise a certain metric such as path length (see, e.g. (Chmarra et al. 2006)). This could lead to the adjustment of a certain task and the choice to use other metrics or to use only expert data to set thresholds.

Contrarily, the application of the theoretic threshold for safe meniscal tissue probing could be used as the absolute maximum value that a trainee might use. Ideally this should be supported by force measurements executed during experiments with real instruments and tissue or by expert data who show probing levels which are all below the theoretic threshold. Especially, since tissue material properties and instrument contact areas used to calculate the forces are not always constant.

As shown in Chaps. 9 and 11, sufficient functional arthroscopic simulators are available as well as metrics to define trainees performance and to monitor progression. The next step is to design and validate sets of training tasks and support there applicability with evidence-based thresholds. The data in this chapter provide the first values that can be used.

Bibliography

Alvand A, Auplish S, Gill H, Rees J (2011) Innate arthroscopic skills in medical students and variation in learning curves. J Bone Joint Surg Am 93(19):e115–e119, available from: PM:22005876

Andersen C, Winding TN, Vesterby MS (2011) Development of simulated arthroscopic skills. Acta Orthop 82(1):90–95, available from: PM:21281257

Buchner M (2009) Aktueller Stand der arthro- skopischen Meniskuschirurgie. Sport Orthopadie Traumatologie 25:171–178

Cannon WD, Nicandri GT, Reinig K, Mevis H, Wittstein J (2014) Evaluation of skill level between trainees and community orthopaedic surgeons using a virtual reality arthroscopic knee simulator. J Bone Joint Surg Am 96(7):e57, available from: PM:24695934

Chmarra MK, Bakker NH, Grimbergen CA, Dankelman J (2006) TrEndo, a device for tracking minimally invasive surgical instruments in training setups. Sensors Actuators A Phys 126(2):328–334, available from: ISI:000235431800007

Cho JH (2014) A modified outside-in suture technique for repair of the middle segment of the meniscus using a spinal needle. Knee Surg Relat Res 26(1):43–47, available from: PM:24639946

Fithian DC, Kelly MA, Mow VC (1990) Material properties and structure-function relationships in the menisci. Clin Orthop Relat Res (252):19–31, available from: PM:2406069

Forkel P, Herbort M, Sprenker F, Metzlaff S, Raschke M, Petersen W (2014) The biomechanical effect of a lateral meniscus posterior root tear with and without damage to the meniscofemoral ligament: efficacy of different repair techniques. Arthroscopy 30:833–840, available from: PM:24780106

Gomoll AH, O'Toole RV, Czarnecki J, Warner JJ (2007) Surgical experience correlates with performance on a virtual reality simulator for shoulder arthroscopy. Am J Sports Med 35(6):883–888, available from: PM:17261572

Heijnsdijk EA, de Visser H, Dankelman J, Gouma DJ (2004) Slip and damage properties of jaws of laparoscopic graspers. Surg Endosc 18(6):974–979, available from: PM:15108111

Howells NR, Brinsden MD, Gill RS, Carr AJ, Rees JL (2008) Motion analysis: a validated method for showing skill levels in arthroscopy. Arthroscopy 24(3):335–342, available from: PM:18308187

Hull ML, Berns GS, Varma H, Patterson HA (1996) Strain in the medial collateral ligament of the human knee under single and combined loads. J Biomech 29(2):199–206, available from: PM:8849813

Kennedy JC, Hawkins RJ, Willis RB, Danylchuck KD (1976) Tension studies of human knee ligaments. Yield point, ultimate failure, and disruption of the cruciate and tibial collateral ligaments. J Bone Joint Surg Am 58(3):350–355, available from: PM:1262366

McCarthy AD, Moody L, Waterworth AR, Bickerstaff DR (2006) Passive haptics in a knee arthroscopy simulator: is it valid for core skills training? Clin Orthop Relat Res 442:13–20, available from: PM:16394733

Meyer M, Graveleau N, Hardy P, Landreau P (2007) Anatomic risks of shoulder arthroscopy portals: anatomic cadaveric study of 12 portals. Arthroscopy 23(5):529–536, available from: PM:17478285

Oxford English Dictionary (2014). Oxford University Press. http://www.oed.com/. Accessed 15 Jan 2014

Pedowitz RA, Esch J, Snyder S (2002) Evaluation of a virtual reality simulator for arthroscopy skills development. Arthroscopy 18(6):E29, available from: PM:12098111

Ra HJ, Ha JK, Jang SH, Lee DW, Kim JG (2013) Arthroscopic inside-out repair of complete radial tears of the meniscus with a fibrin clot. Knee Surg Sports Traumatol Arthrosc 21(9):2126–2130, available from: PM:23000919

Robinson JR, Bull AM, Amis AA (2005) Structural properties of the medial collateral ligament complex of the human knee. J Biomech 38(5):1067–1074, available from: PM:15797588

Rodrigues SP, Horeman T, Dankelman J, van den Dobbelsteen JJ, Jansen FW (2012) Suturing intra-abdominal organs: when do we cause tissue damage? Surg Endosc 26(4):1005–1009, available from: PM:22028014

Schreuder HW, van Hove PD, Janse JA, Verheijen RR, Stassen LP, Dankelman J (2011) An "intermediate curriculum" for advanced laparoscopic skills training with virtual reality simulation. J Minim Invasive Gynecol 18(5):597–606, available from: PM:21783431

Soubeyrand M, Bauer T, Billot N, Lortat-Jacob A, Gicquelet R, Hardy P (2008) Original portals for arthroscopic decompression of the suprascapular nerve: an anatomic study. J Shoulder Elbow Surg 17(4):616–623, available from: PM:18276165

Stunt JJ, Wulms PH, Kerkhoffs GM, Sierevelt IN, Schafroth MU, Tuijthof GJ (2013) Variation in joint stressing magnitudes during knee arthroscopy. Knee Surg Sports Traumatol Arthrosc, available from: PM:23740322

Tashiro Y, Miura H, Nakanishi Y, Okazaki K, Iwamoto Y (2009) Evaluation of skills in arthroscopic training based on trajectory and force data. Clin Orthop Relat Res 467(2):546–552, available from: PM:18791774

Trent PS, Walker PS, Wolf B (1976) Ligament length patterns, strength, and rotational axes of the knee joint. Clin Orthop Relat Res (117):263–270, available from: PM:1277674

Tuijthof GJ, Meulman HN, Herder JL, van Dijk CN (2009) Meniscal shear stress for punching. J Appl Biomater Biomech 7(2):97–103, available from: PM:20799169

Tuijthof GJ, van Sterkenburg MN, Sierevelt IN, Van OJ, van Dijk CN, Kerkhoffs GM (2010) First validation of the PASSPORT training environment for arthroscopic skills. Knee Surg Sports Traumatol Arthrosc 18(2):218–224, available from: PM:19629441

Tuijthof GJ, Horeman T, Schafroth MU, Blankevoort L, Kerkhoffs GM (2011) Probing forces of menisci: what levels are safe for arthroscopic surgery. Knee Surg Sports Traumatol Arthrosc 19(2):248–254, available from: PM:20814661

Monitoring Performance and Progression in the Operating Theatre

13

Gabriëlle J.M. Tuijthof and Inger N. Sierevelt

Take-Home Messages

- The definition of standardised benchmarks is required to define arthroscopic competency.
- Measuring surgical performance comes with challenges, but new developments such as affordable tracking systems and video analysis software can facilitate structural implementation.
- Objective monitoring of resident learning curves is feasible using global rating scales.
- ASSET and BAKSSS global rating scales are validated most extensively and suggested to be used in clinical practice, where ASSET offers potential for summative assessment of arthroscopic skills.

13.1 Introduction

Although previous chapters indicated the potential and benefits of training arthroscopic skills in simulated environments, training needs to be

G.J.M. Tuijthof (✉)
Department of Biomechanical Engineering, Delft University of Technology, Delft, The Netherlands

Department of Orthopedic Surgery, Academic Medical Centre, Amsterdam, The Netherlands
e-mail: g.j.m.tuijthof@tudelft.nl

I.N. Sierevelt, MSc
Department of Orthopedics, Slotervaart Hospital, Amsterdam, The Netherlands
e-mail: i.sierevelt@gmail.com

continued in the operating room to achieve the necessary proficiency. Based on the theory on learning strategies in Chap. 4, it is posed that if residents indeed acquire the basic skills before they enter the operating room, the focus in the operating room can be on more complex tasks. This requires the formulation of guidelines that determine the level that qualifies proficiency. For the actual cases in the operating room, this is a difficult task as the level of complexity of the procedure plays an important role, and proficiency is not necessarily defined as the summation of several part-task skills, but rather requires a holistic approach.

Generally, the complexity of an arthroscopy is divided in two levels: basic (removal) and advanced (reconstruction), e.g. meniscectomy vs. anterior cruciate ligament (ACL) reconstruction (Morris et al. 1993; O'Neill et al. 2002). For elbow arthroscopy, five levels of complexity have been defined (Savoie 2007). To cope with the complexity and support the holistic judgment, faculty members from recognised institutions that have performed a substantial number of procedures (>250) themselves qualify to judge proficiency (Morris et al. 1993; O'Neill et al. 2002) – a method that is being applied in many residency curricula. Despite arthroscopy being performed frequently, consensus is to be attained on the exact definition of arthroscopic competence and the number of procedures that are required to achieve it (Hodgins and Veillette 2013; O'Neill et al. 2002).

M. Karahan et al. (eds.), *Effective Training of Arthroscopic Skills*,
DOI 10.1007/978-3-662-44943-1_13, © ESSKA 2015

As little to no evidence is available on transfer validity of arthroscopic simulator training, and many residency curricula have yet to implement simulator training, the first section focuses on measuring surgical performance in the operating theatre. Measuring surgical performance is not only useful in training, but has also direct applications in quantification and monitoring of operative quality, patient safety and workflow optimisation. Tools and methods are presented from these areas. These could be applied to verify proficiency in basic arthroscopic skills. Additionally, work is presented to set reference baselines for comparing surgical performance.

As mentioned, training in the OR consists of the apprentice model, where the resident initially watches the teaching surgeon performing an operation and gradually takes over (Pedowitz et al. 2002). As modern medicine offers reduced time for residents to develop their arthroscopic skills, it is worthwhile to optimise the learning effect per operation. General educational theories indicate that feedback on one's performance and stimulation of active learning contributes significantly to a more effective learning process (Prince 2004). For surgery, it has been demonstrated that direct feedback on performance improves the resident's individual skills (Harewood et al. 2008; O'Connor et al. 2008). We present tools that are suitable to monitor this form of teaching and respect the holistic judgment model needed to assess the more complex tasks.

13.2 Measuring Surgical Performance and Baseline References

Measuring surgical performance is not an easy task, as patient care has number one priority, patient privacy and the sterile operating zone should be respected, and the operating theatre cannot be transformed into an experimental set-up. Besides, interpretation of the data is complex. That is why attention is paid as well to the registration of baseline reference data of procedures currently performed in the operating theatre. Two categories of tools are defined: sensors that can

measure psychomotor skills similarly as done in simulated environments and video and audio registrations that can capture overall surgical performance. Each is elucidated with examples.

13.2.1 Sensors

The first parameter to be discussed is not surprisingly the operation time. It is easy to measure and often used to track operative planning and workflow. Its value is deducted from the well-established fact that experts execute surgical actions more efficiently compared to novices (Bridges and Diamond 1999). Farnworth and co-workers demonstrated that residents are significantly slower in performing ACL reconstructions compared to orthopaedic surgeons, which can also have financial consequences (Farnworth et al. 2001).

Psychomotor skills can also be monitored in the operating theatre by motion-tracking systems. Such systems exist using (infrared) cameras that track optical or reflective markers attached to the hands of the surgeon or the instruments or of electromagnetic systems with active markers. In surgical practice, such tracking systems are commonly used in computer-aided surgery for accurate positioning of orthopaedic implants (Fig. 13.1) (Matziolis et al. 2007; Moon et al. 2012; Rosenberger et al. 2008). Tracking can also be performed with normal video cameras and digital image-processing tools that recognise markers or other features in the image. Examples are presented by Doignon and co-workers (Blum et al. 2010; Doignon et al. 2005) who detected surgical instruments in the endoscopic video based on metal-coloured features of the system and by Bouarfa and co-workers who labelled various instruments with coloured markers at the tip to improve robustness (Fig. 13.2) (Bouarfa et al. 2012). Tracking of instrument motions provides insight in surgical performance and flow of the procedure (Aggarwal et al. 2007; Dosis et al. 2005). It does require careful data interpretation.

Another set of parameters that have been measured in the operating room are the forces and

Fig. 13.1 Example of an infrared camera tracking system used in combination with passive reflective markers. (**a**) Infrared camera. (**b**) Two markers attached to the shaft of (**c**) The arthroscopic punch. (**d**) Anatomic bench model of the knee joint (© GJM Tuijthof, 2014. Reprinted with permission)

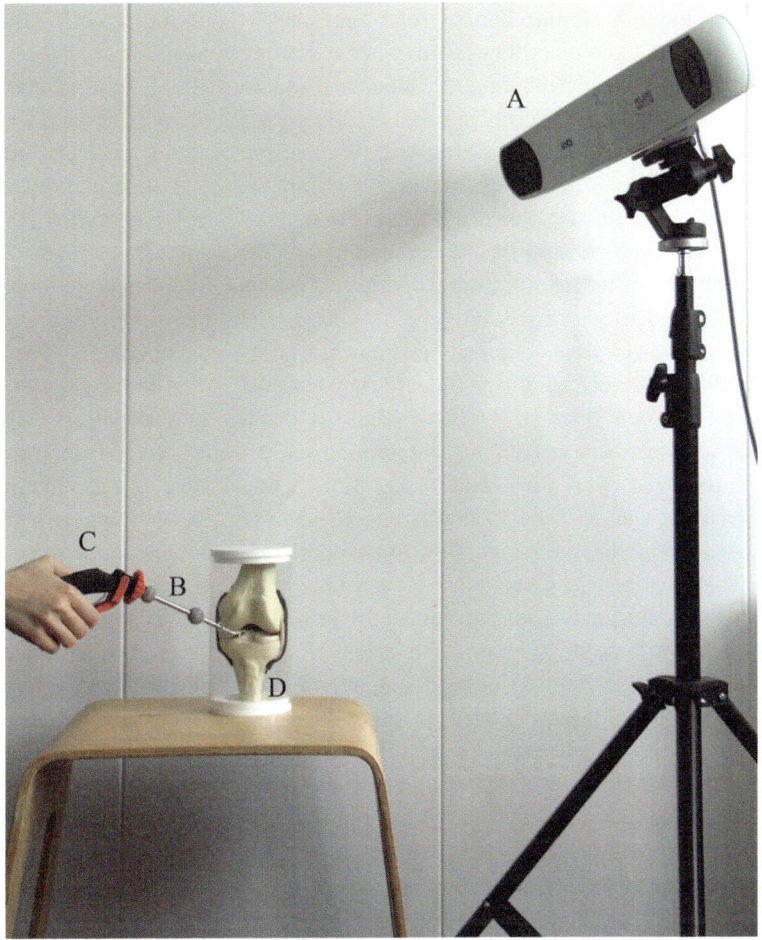

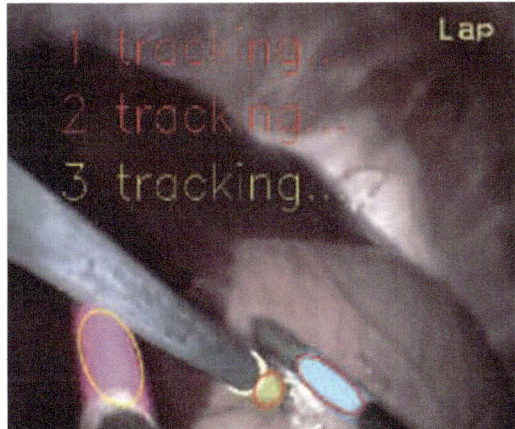

Fig. 13.2 Example of real-time in vivo instrument tracking using coloured labels attached to instruments. In this example three instruments are tracked simultaneously (Bouarfa et al. (2012), copyright © 2012, Informa Healthcare. Reproduced with permission of Informa Healthcare)

torques executed during knee arthroscopy (Chami et al. 2006). Chami and co-workers showed that force parameters can indeed discriminate between novices and experts (Chami et al. 2008).

13.2.2 Video and Audio

Video recordings of a procedure could offer a tool which allows a holistic type of feedback with easy interpretative illustrations. However, the few studies that we could find on using video feedback to improve surgical training did not find significant differences (Backstein et al. 2004; Backstein et al. 2005). Drawbacks of using video recordings are that the replay of an entire operation is time-consuming and without post-processing they do not provide objective measures. A similar line of reasoning can be given for audio recordings. Still, when executing post-processing techniques, video and audio recordings reveal useful cues that could be used to monitor surgical performance. We present some examples related to arthroscopic training.

Time-action analysis is a quantitative method to determine the number and duration of actions. It represents the relative timing of different events and the duration of the individual events. In the medical field, time-action analysis has proven its value in objectifying and quantifying surgical actions (den Boer et al. 2002; Minekus et al. 2003; Sjoerdsma et al. 2000). For training, patient safety and workflow monitoring, time-action analysis can be used to detect and to analyse deviations from the normal flow of the operation. This requires documentation of reference data sets through analysis of procedures performed by expert orthopaedic surgeons. We have performed such analyses for a set of predominantly menis-cectomies with the intended purpose of investi-gating the effectiveness of arthroscopic pump systems (Tuijthof et al. 2007, 2008). To do so, the operations were divided into four phases – (1) creation of portals, (2) joint inspection with or without a probe, (3) cutting and (4) shaving – and their share in the operation time was quantified with the time-action analysis. Comparing the mean duration of each of the phases with those of a trainee can indicate if the trainee performs according to normal workflow or needs substan-tially more time for a certain phase. By analysing the number of instrument exchanges, repeated actions or the percentage of disturbed arthroscopic view as well, trainees can receive detailed objective feedback on the skills they need to improve. Other parameters that were analysed are the prevalence of instrument loss, triangula-tion time and prevalence of lookdowns, which showed a high correlation with global rating scale and motion analysis (Alvand et al. 2012).

As these early time-action analyses initially were performed manually by replaying the video frame by frame (den Boer et al. 2002; Minekus et al. 2003; Sjoerdsma et al. 2000; Tuijthof et al. 2007, 2008), implementation of this method for training purposes is unrealistic as it is too time-consuming. However, efforts have been made to

perform such analyses automatically using image-processing techniques (Doignon et al. 2005; Tuijthof et al. 2011) or specific tracking systems (Bouarfa et al. 2012). When combined with statistical models, such as Markov models, one can even predict peroperatively what the flow of the operation is (Bouarfa et al. 2011; Bouarfa and Dankelman 2012; Padoy et al. 2012). Such methods could lead to tools that provide real-time objective feedback to a trainee during the operation.

Another feasible approach to implement time-action analysis techniques for training purposes is derived from training of high performance ath-letes. In this field, it is becoming a daily practice that training activities are recorded on video. To cope with the huge amount of data, sports analy-sis video software has been developed, which makes it easier to tag events, to assign event to categories, to make annotations and to perform quantitative analyses. Examples of commercial video analysis software packages are Utilius (CCC software, Leipzig, Germany, www.ccc-software.de), MotionView™ (AllSportSystems, Willow Springs, USA, www.allsportsystems.com) and SportsCode Gamebreaker Plus (Sportstec, Sydney, Australia, www.sportstec.com). We present an example of applying such software for the analysis of verbal feedback during arthroscopic training in our university hospital. During supervised training of arthros-copy, verbal communication is mainly used to guide the resident through the procedure. This suggests that the training process can be moni-tored through verbal communication. To investi-gate if current training in the operating room involves sufficient feedback and/or questioning to stimulate active learning, verbal communica-tion was objectified and quantified.

Within a period of two times 3 months, 18 arthroscopic knee procedures were recorded with a special capturing system consisting of two video cameras – one from the arthroscopic camera and one of the hands of the residents (digital CCD camera, 21CW, Sony CCD, Tokyo, Japan) – and a tie-clip microphone (ECM-3003, Monacor, Bremen, Germany) that was mounted on the supervising surgeon. The video images were combined by a colour quad proces-

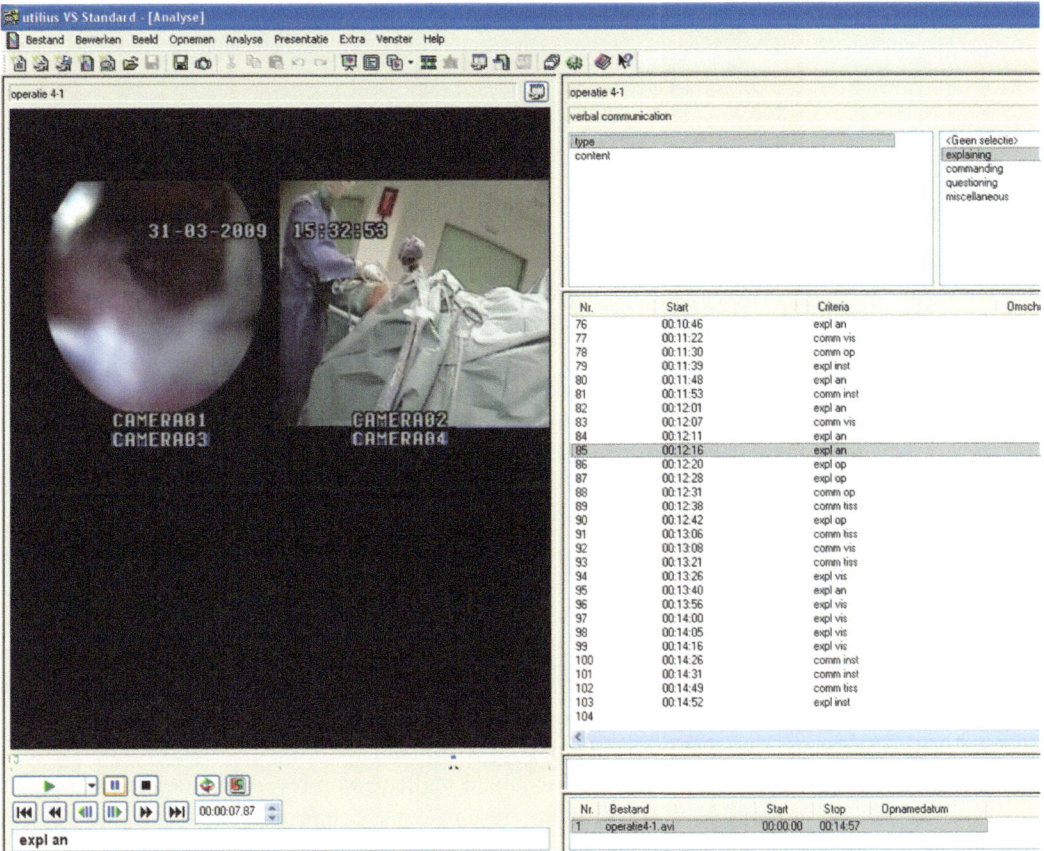

Fig. 13.3 Screenshot of software used to analyse verbal communication (© GJM Tuijthof, 2014. Reprinted with permission)

sor (GS-C4CQR, Golden State Instrument Co., Tustin, USA) and digitised simultaneously with the sound by an A/D converter (ADVC 110, GV Thomson, Paris, France). Four residents who were supervised by either one of two participating surgeons performed the operations. Communication events were tagged with Utilius VS 4.3.2 (CCC-software, Leipzig, Germany) and assigned to categories for the type and content of communication (Fig. 13.3). Four communication types were adopted from Blom et al. (2007): explaining, questioning, commanding and miscellaneous (Table 13.1). As this study specifically focuses on training, one category was added, feedback, which reflects the judgment of the teaching surgeon on the actions of the resident. Six categories for communication content were defined as follows: operation method (that has an accent on steps that have to be taken in the near future e.g. start creating the second portal), anat-

omy and pathology, instrument handling and tissue interaction (e.g. open punch, reposition instrument, stress joint, increase portal size, push meniscus backwards), visualisation (e.g. move scope, irrigation, focus), miscellaneous (general or private) and indefinable (Table 13.1). The frequency of events as percentage of total events in each of the categories was determined (Table 13.1). A multivariable linear regression analysis was performed to determine if the teaching surgeon and the experience of the residents significantly influenced the frequency of communication events per minute ($p<0.05$).

On average 6.0 (SD 1.8) communication events took place every minute. The communication types *explaining* and *commanding* show a considerable frequency compared to *questioning* and *feedback* (Table 13.1). The explaining events were primarily on *anatomy and pathology* followed by *instrument handling and tissue interac-*

Table 13.1 Crosstabs for type (upper row) and content (left column) categories as percentage of total events

	Total (%)	Explaining (%)	Commanding (%)	Questioning (%)	Feedback (%)	Miscellaneous (%)
Total	100.0	38.8	27.4	5.7	10.6	17.4
Operation method	4.2	3.6	0.1	0.1	0.5	0.0
Anatomy and pathology	17.7	14.8	0.0	2.4	0.5	0.0
Instrument handling and tissue interaction	35.7	13.0	14.2	2.0	6.4	0.1
Visualisation	24.9	7.4	13.1	1.2	3.2	0.0
Miscellaneous	14.0	0.0	0.1	0.1	0.0	13.9
Indefinable	3.5	0.0	0.0	0.0	0.0	3.5

tion. The commanding events were primarily on *instrument handling and tissue interaction* and *visualisation*, which in general were the most frequent communication content categories (Table 13.1). A difference in mean events per minute was found between both teaching surgeons ($p < 0.05$). No significant correlation was found between the frequency of events and the experience of the residents.

The results highlight distinctive communication patterns. The relative high frequency of the types *explaining* and *commanding* as opposed to *questioning* and *feedback* is noticeable as the latter two stimulate active learning in general. Additionally, explaining on the contents *anatomy and pathology* and *instrument handling and tissue interaction* is considerable. These items are particularly suitable for training outside the operating room. If trained so, more options are left to focus on other learning goals. As a clear difference was present between the frequency of events per minute amongst the surgeons and no correlation was found for the experience of residents, we cannot confirm that this method is suitable as an objective evaluation tool for new training methods. Additional research is recommended with a larger group of residents to minimise the effect of outliers.

13.3 Monitoring Complex Tasks and Assessing Learning Curves

To respect the holistic assessment model, expert surgeons are needed to assess the more complex tasks. This type of assessment is sensitive to the subjective opinion of the assessor, which might compromise fair judgment (Mabrey et al. 2002). To overcome this issue, education theories recommend the formulation of rubrics, which describe clear evaluation criteria and various levels of competence. In surgical training, such rubrics are called global rating scales (GRS). The GRS suggested that arthroscopic skills will be elucidated as well as their validation and examples to assess learning curves.

Within this section, we loosely follow Hodgins and Veillette who reviewed assessment tools for arthroscopic competency (Hodgins and Veillette 2013). Recently, various GRS have been developed specifically for structured, objective feedback during training of arthroscopies (Table 13.2):

1. Orthopaedic Competence Assessment Project (OCAP) (Howells et al. 2008)
2. Basic Arthroscopic Knee Skill Scoring System (BAKSSS) (Insel et al. 2009)
3. Arthroscopic Skills Assessment (ASA) (Elliott et al. 2012)
4. Objective Assessment of Arthroscopic Skills (OAAS) (Slade Shantz et al. 2013)
5. Arthroscopic Surgery Skill Evaluation Tool (ASSET) (Koehler et al. 2013)

The actual forms are available in Appendices 13.A, 13.B, 13.C, 13.D and 13.E. Noticeable is that all arthroscopic GRS except for ASA have a similar structure with 7–10 items that need to be scored on a 5-point Likert scale. At least 3 of 5 points are explicitly described, which should help uniform assessment. Also

Table 13.2 All GRS that are suggested for rating of arthroscopic skills based on Hodgins and Veillette (2013)

Acronyms of Global Rating Scales	Description	Validation
OCAP	9 items, scored on a 1–5 point Likert scale	Based on OSATS validation protocols
BAKSSS	10 items, scored on a 1–5 point Likert scale	Construct validity level of experience ($p<0.05$)
		Concurrent validity with year of residency ($r=0.93$)
		Concurrent validity with motion analysis ($r=0.58$) (Alvand et al. 2013)
		Internal consistency (Cronbach's $\alpha=0.88$) (Alvand et al. 2013)
		Interrater reliability (kappa$=0.543$) (Olson et al. 2013)
ASA	100-point score, 75 for structure identification, 25 for time to completion and penalties for cartilage damage	Construct validity level of experience ($p<0.001$)
OAAS	7 items, scored on a 1–5 point Likert scale, complexity of procedure	Construct validity level of experience ($p<0.0001$)
		Internal consistency (Cronbach's $\alpha=0.97$)
		Level of agreement (ICC$=0.80$)
		Test-retest reliability ($r=0.52$)
ASSET	8 items, scored on a 1–5 point Likert scale, complexity of procedure	Content validity: expert group
		Concurrent validity level of experience ($p<0.05$)
		Level of agreement (ICC$=0.90$)
		Test-retest reliability ($r=0.79$)

The forms can be found in Appendices 13.A, 13.B, 13.C, 13.D and 13.E

many of the items are similar, such as instrument handling, flow of operation, efficiency and autonomy. OCAP and BAKSSS are also recommended to be used with task-specific checklists, whereas ASA solely focuses on knee arthroscopy with such a checklist. Analysing these GRS, one can conclude that a certain level of consensus exists on arthroscopic skills that a resident should be able to demonstrate in the operating theatre and the required level to qualify as competent.

OCAP is not specifically tested, but its items are derived from the well-established OSATS GRS, which has been validated extensively (Martin et al. 1997; Reznick et al. 1997). The four other GRS have been validated for construct, content and concurrent validity as well as internal consistency, interrater and test-retest reliability (Table 13.2). The results indicate that they meet the requirements and show a high correlation with year of residency. Notice that none of the study designs for validation are the same, thus one-to-one comparison is not possible. The

ASSET has also been evaluated for summative assessment in a pass-fail examination, which was confirmed with a high rater agreement (ICC$=0.83$) (Koehler and Nicandri 2013).

For OCAP and BAKSSS, we determined if they reflect the learning curve during arthroscopic training in the operating room and what their discriminative level is. 75 arthroscopic procedures performed by 15 residents in their fourth, fifth and sixth year of their residency were assessed by their supervising surgeon.

Pearson correlation coefficients were calculated between year of residence and normalised sum scores of both GRS questionnaires. The normalised sum score consisted of all points scored on each of the items normalised to a 100-point scale. The Pearson correlation was significant for BAKSSS ($R=0.73$) and for OCAP 0.70 ($R=0.70$). A linear regression analysis demonstrated a significant increase of the GRS sum score of 9.2 points (95 % CI 6.2–12.1) for BAKSSS and 9.5 points (95 % CI 6.5–12.5) for

OCAP. The results lead to our conclusion that both GRS are suitable to monitor overall arthroscopic skills progression in the operating theatre.

Now that the tools for monitoring surgical performance in the operating theatre are summarised, this section focusses on the application of these tools to assess learning curves. As the number of studies is quite limited all are briefly described. The learning curve of arthroscopic rotator cuff repair was determined using operation time as metric (Guttmann et al. 2005). Using blocks of ten operations for comparison, a significant decrease in operation was determined between the first two blocks, but not for consecutive blocks. This indicates that learning took place in the first ten procedures. The learning curve for hip arthroscopy is determined by measuring the operation but also by determining the complication rate (Hoppe et al. 2014). Improvement was seen between early and late experience with 30 patient cases as being the most common cut-off. A similar study design was used to assess the learning curve for arthroscopic Latarjet procedures, which showed a significant decrease in operation time and complication rate between the first 15 patient cases and the consecutive 15 patient cases (Castricini et al. 2013). Van Oldenrijk and co-workers, who used time-action analysis to assess a learning curve for minimally invasive total hip arthroplasty, found that learning took place in the first five to ten patient cases (Van Oldenrijk et al. 2008). This was quantified by the number of repetitions, waiting and additional actions executed during the operation.

13.4 Discussion

In this chapter, monitoring tools to measure surgical performance and training progression were presented. Operation time is easy to measure and as shown capable of reflecting learning curves. Still, using the operation time as a measure for training purposes is less useful, since it does not give clues for the trainee on what to improve, and it reflects many more factors than the surgical

performance such as the complexity of the patient case. This is also acknowledged in the global rating scales. The tracking systems that have been used on research studies are quite expensive and require preoperative installation and calibration, which could explain the absence of studies performed in the operating room to determine learning curves. However, in the entertainment and gaming industry, motion-tracking developments are growing fast, from which the surgical training field could benefit. For example, Wii controllers are affordable and their accuracy is continuously being improved. Measuring of forces as presented by Chami requires a specific measurement set-up and modification of the instruments (Chami et al. 2008). Furthermore, attention needs to be paid on the manner of feedback using force parameters as the feedback should make sense for the trainee. Overall, these metrics are used in simulated environments and are strong in monitoring confined less complex tasks or actions. However, video monitoring seems to reflect the required holistic judgment model needed to assess more complex cognitive tasks. The challenge is to cope with the huge amounts of data that video registration gives. In that perspective, automatic detection with image-based tracking algorithms would be a perfect alternative tool as the arthroscopic view is available anyhow. However, until now these algorithms lacked robustness due to continuous changing lighting conditions in the view. With this feature perspective, video analysis software as applied in athlete training might be a good alternative at short notice, especially if supervising surgeons define critical phases of the procedure that will be the focus of the learning experience, since this would limit the video recordings to those events solely. A major advantage of video analysis is that it can provided highly comprehensive feedback to the trainee. Another alternative is the use of global rating scales. These scales structure and objectify the feedback of the supervising surgeons, but cannot be so illustrative as video feedback. Furthermore, it is recommended that assessors using the scales are trained to attain uniform assessment. However, they are truly easy to implement in residency curricula, have been demonstrated to reflect the learning curve of residents and could also be used for self-assessment. Summarizing, quite some tools have been presented, and validation of GRS for arthroscopic skills has been performed. This offers feasible tools to continue arthroscopic skills monitoring in an objective, structured and comprehensive manner that is formative assessment. Still more research is required to determine which of the tools could be used for summative assessment.

13.5   Appendix 13.A Orthopaedic Competence Assessment Project

Skill	Score 1	Score 2	Score 3	Score 4	Score 5
Follows protocol	Unsatisfactory		Adequate. Occasional need for guidance and help		Excellent adherence to agreed protocol. No prompts. No mistakes
Handles tissue well	Careless. Potential to cause damage		Adequate. No tissue damage. Occasional need for increased care		Excellent tissue handling. Precise and delicate
Appropriate and safe use of instruments	Dangerous. Risk to patient and assistant. Potential for damage to equipment		Adequate use of instruments and scope. Occasional guidance to ensure instruments remain within field of vision		Excellent use of instruments. Good control of arthroscope. Instruments constantly within field of vision
Appropriate pace with economy of movement	Erratic pace and movements. Overly rushing or inappropriately slow		Adequate economy of movement. Majority of movements controlled and careful. Occasional erratic movement		Excellent fluidity and economy of movement. Procedure performed at appropriate pace without erratic movements
Act calmly and effectively with untoward events	Unable to deal with adverse events. Panic and inability to respond		Remains calm. Remains safe. Takes advice from supervisor. Unable to cope independently		Excellent ability to cope with adverse events. Remains calm. Deals with complication independently
Appropriate use of assistant	Fails to involve assistant appropriately. Resultant poor positioning. Poor rapport		Asks for appropriate joint position at appropriate times. Unable to suggest alternative positions to improve view/access		Excellent use of assistant. Good rapport. Able to constantly modify input of assistant to best advantage throughout procedure
Communicates with scrubs nurse	Inappropriate communication resulting in confusion or operative delay		Appropriate communication with scrub nurse. Occasional need for clarification from supervisor		Excellent rapport with scrub nurse. Clear and effective communication, maximising procedural efficiency
Clearly identifies common abnormalities	Unable to identify common abnormalities. Confusion over basic anatomy		Adequate identification of common pathology. Occasional mistake. Unsure of precise classifications		Excellent knowledge of pathology of common abnormalities. Clear understanding of classification of injuries

Skill	Score 1	Score 2	Score 3	Score 4	Score 5
Protecting the articular surface	Inability to protect articular surface appropriately. Potential to cause damage		Awareness of need to protect articular surface. Adequate care taken. Occasional prompt from supervisor required		Excellent awareness of articular surfaces. High degree of care maintained throughout the procedure

13.6 Appendix 13.B Basic Arthroscopic Knee Skill Scoring System

Skill	Score 1	Score 2	Score 3	Score 4	Score 5
Dissection	Appeared excessively hesitant, caused trauma to tissues, did not dissect into correct anatomical plan		Controlled and safe dissection into correct anatomical plane, caused minimal trauma to tissues		Superior and atraumatic dissection into the correct anatomical plane
Instrument handling	Repeatedly makes tentative or awkward movements with instruments		Competent use of instruments, although occasionally appeared stuff or awkward		Fluid moves with instruments and no awkwardness
Depth perception	Constantly overshoots target, slow to correct		Some overshooting or missing of target		Accurately directs instruments in the correct plane to target
Bimanual dexterity	Noticeably awkward with non-dominant hand, poor coordination between hands		Uses both hands but does not maximise interaction between hands		Expertly uses both hands in complementary manner to provide optimum performance
Flow of operation and forward planning	Frequently stopped operating or needed to discuss next move		Demonstrated ability for forward planning with steady progression of operative procedure		Obviously planned course of operation with effortless flow from one move to the next
Knowledge of instruments	Frequently asked for the wrong instrument or used inappropriate instrument		Knew the names of most instruments and used appropriate instrument for the task		Obviously familiar with the instruments required and their names
Efficiency	Many unnecessary, inefficient movements. Constantly changing focus or persisting without progress		Slow, but planned movements are reasonably organised with few unnecessary or repetitive movements		Confident, clear economy of movement and maximum efficiency
Knowledge of specific procedure	Deficient knowledge, needed specific instruction at most operative steps		Knew all important aspects of the operation		Demonstrated familiarity with all aspects of the operation
Autonomy	Unable to complete entire task, even with verbal guidance		Able to complete task safely with moderate guidance		Able to complete task independently without prompting
Quality of final product	Very poor		Competent		Clearly superior

13.7   Appendix 13.C Arthroscopic Skills Assessment

Start time	Stop time	Total time
Landmark	To be visualised	Score
Suprapatellar pouch	View all areas of pouch	(3)
Patella	View medial facet	(3)
	View lateral facets	(3)
Trochlea	View trochlear surface	(4)
Medical recess	View medial gutter/assess meniscal synovial junction	(4)
Lateral recess	View lateral gutter/assess meniscal junction/popliteus	(4)
Medial compartment	Assess condyle for chondral lesions	(5)
	Meniscus/view anterior, middle, posterior	(5)
	Probe superior and inferior surface	(10)
Intercondylar notch	View and inspect ACL	(5)
	View and inspect PCL	(5)
Lateral compartment	Assess condyle for chondral lesions	(5)
	Meniscus/view anterior, middle, posterior	(5)
	Probe superior and inferior surface	(10)
	View popliteus tendon	(4)

	Missed items	Scope score
Time	Time penalty	Total time score
		Total score

13.8   Appendix 13.D Objective Assessment of Arthroscopic Skills

Skill	Novice	Advanced beginner	Competent	Proficient	Expert
Examining/ manipulating joint	Did not examine joint or position to give improved visualisation during procedure	Examined joint without diagnostic abilities and lacked ability to facilitate view by positioning	Positioned knee appropriately after some difficulty with visualisation	Used common positioning to facilitate view during arthroscopy	Used accepted and novel positioning to perform the arthroscopy effortlessly
Triangulating instruments	Could not insert instruments into ports and maintain them in view. Unable to locate instrument tips without difficulty	Unable to maintain instrument in field of view consistently	Found instruments with delay. Field of view wandered from operative site but returned	Found instruments quickly and began work. Occasionally delayed in orienting camera to afford better visualisation	Immediately located instruments and began work without delay. Kept instrument in field of view at all times
Controlling fluid flow and joint distension	Under-/ overdistended joint consistently due to inappropriate matching of suction and flow.	Achieved proper distension after delays. Some extravasation into tissue due to overdistension	Distended joint adequately after initial loss of pressure during suction	Joint distended appropriately through control of flow and suction	Minimal fluid extravasated with constantly maintained field of view

Skill	Novice	Advanced beginner	Competent	Proficient	Expert
Maintaining field of view	Often disoriented. Was unable to adjust scope to improve visualisation	Maintained field of view part of the time	Maintained and adjusted arthroscope to provide maximal view with some difficulty	Maintained field of view in same portal	Changed portals quickly to improve visualisation
Controlling instruments	Was unable to perform tasks with provided instruments. Caused cartilage damage	Repeatedly made tentative or awkward moves with instruments	Competently used instruments although occasionally appeared stiff or awkward	Used instruments appropriately and efficiently	Made fluid moves with instruments and used some instruments in novel ways to increase efficiency
Economising time and planning forward	Was unable to complete any portion of the procedure	Was able to complete components of the procedure, but needed to discuss next move	Completed all components of the operation with some unnecessary moves	Was efficient, but continued discovering new time saving motions	Showed economy of movement and maximum efficiency
Overall	Possessed rudimentary arthroscopic skills with only basic anatomical and mechanical understanding	Knew basic steps of procedure and performed some independently	Performed the procedure independently	Performed procedure with changes to improve efficiency	Performed the procedure with minimal chance to improve efficiency
Complexity	No difficulties	Slightly difficult	Moderately difficult	Considerable difficulty	Critical

13.9   Appendix 13.E Arthroscopic Surgical Skill Evaluation Tool

Skill	Score 1	Score 2	Score 3	Score 4	Score 5
Safety	Significant damage to articular cartilage or soft tissue		Insignificant damage to articular cartilage or soft tissue		No damage to articular cartilage or soft tissue
Field of view	Narrow field of view, inadequate arthroscope or light source positioning		Moderate field of view, adequate arthroscope and light source positioning		Expansive field of view, optimal arthroscope and light source positioning
Camera dexterity	Awkward or graceless movements, fails to keep camera centred and correctly oriented		Appropriate use of camera, occasionally needs to reposition		Graceful and dexterous throughout procedure with camera always centred and correctly
Instrument dexterity	Overly tentative or awkward with instruments, unable to consistently direct instruments to targets		Careful, controlled use of instruments, occasionally misses targets		Confident and accurate use of all instruments

Skill	Score 1	Score 2	Score 3	Score 4	Score 5
Bimanual dexterity	Unable to use both hands or no coordination between hands		Uses both hands but occasionally fails to coordinate movement of camera and instruments		Uses both hands to coordinate camera and instrument positioning for optimal performance
Flow of procedure	Frequently stops operating or persists without progress, multiple unsuccessful attempts prior to completing tasks		Steady progression of operative procedure with few unsuccessful attempts prior to completing tasks		Obviously planned course of procedure, fluid transition from one task to the next with no unsuccessful attempts
Quality of procedure	Inadequate or incomplete final product		Adequate final product with only minor flaws that do not require correction		Optimal final product with no flaws
Autonomy	Unable to complete procedure even with intervention(s)		Able to complete procedure but required intervention(s)		Able to complete procedure without intervention
Complexity	No difficulty		Moderate difficulty (mild inflammation or scarring)		Extreme difficulty (severe inflammation or scarring, abnormal anatomy)

Bibliography

Aggarwal R, Grantcharov T, Moorthy K, Milland T, Papasavas P, Dosis A, Bello F, Darzi A (2007) An evaluation of the feasibility, validity, and reliability of laparoscopic skills assessment in the operating room. Ann Surg 245(6):992–999, available from: PM:17522527

Alvand A, Khan T, Al-Ali S, Jackson WF, Price AJ, Rees JL (2012) Simple visual parameters for objective assessment of arthroscopic skill. J Bone Joint Surg Am 94(13):e97, available from: PM:22760398

Alvand A, Logishetty K, Middleton R, Khan T, Jackson WF, Price AJ, Rees JL (2013) Validating a global rating scale to monitor individual resident learning curves during arthroscopic knee meniscal repair. Arthroscopy 29(5):906–912, available from: PM:23628663

Backstein D, Agnidis Z, Regehr G, Reznick R (2004) The effectiveness of video feedback in the acquisition of orthopedic technical skills. Am J Surg 187(3):427–432, available from: PM:15006577

Backstein D, Agnidis Z, Sadhu R, MacRae H (2005) Effectiveness of repeated video feedback in the acquisition of a surgical technical skill. Can J Surg 48(3):195–200, available from: PM:16013622

Blom EM, Verdaasdonk EG, Stassen LP, Stassen HG, Wieringa PA, Dankelman J (2007) Analysis of verbal communication during teaching in the operating room and the potentials for surgical training. Surg Endosc 21(9):1560–1566, available from: PM:17285367

Blum T, Feussner H, Navab N (2010) Modeling and segmentation of surgical workflow from laparoscopic video. Med Image Comput Comput Assist Interv 13(Pt 3):400–407, available from: PM:20879425

Bouarfa L, Akman O, Schneider A, Jonker PP, Dankelman J (2012) In-vivo real-time tracking of surgical instruments in endoscopic video. Minim Invasive Ther Allied Technol 21(3):129–134, available from: PM:21574828

Bouarfa L, Dankelman J (2012) Workflow mining and outlier detection from clinical activity logs. J Biomed Inform 45(6):1185–1190, available from: PM:22925724

Bouarfa L, Jonker PP, Dankelman J (2011) Discovery of high-level tasks in the operating room. J Biomed Inform 44(3):455–462, available from: PM:20060495

Bridges M, Diamond DL (1999) The financial impact of teaching surgical residents in the operating room. Am J Surg 177(1):28–32, available from: PM:10037304

Castricini R, De Benedetto M, Orlando N, Rocchi M, Zini R, Pirani P (2013) Arthroscopic Latarjet procedure: analysis of the learning curve. Musculoskelet Surg 97(Suppl 1):93–98, available from: PM:23588833

Chami G, Ward J, Wills D, Phillips R, Sherman K (2006) Smart tool for force measurements during knee arthroscopy: in vivo human study. Stud Health Technol Inform 119:85–89, available from: PM:16404020

Chami G, Ward JW, Phillips R, Sherman KP (2008) Haptic feedback can provide an objective assessment of arthroscopic skills. Clin Orthop Relat Res 466(4):963–968, available from: PM:18213507

den Boer KT, Bruijn M, Jaspers JE, Stassen LP, Erp WF, Jansen A, Go PM, Dankelman J, Gouma DJ (2002)

Time-action analysis of instrument positioners in laparoscopic cholecystectomy. Surg Endosc 16(1):142–147, available from: PM:11961625

Doignon C, Graebling P, de Mathelin M (2005) Real-time segmentation of surgical instruments inside the abdominal cavity using a joint hue saturation color feature. Real Time Imaging 11:429–442

Dosis A, Aggarwal R, Bello F, Moorthy K, Munz Y, Gillies D, Darzi A (2005) Synchronized video and motion analysis for the assessment of procedures in the operating theater. Arch Surg 140:293–299

Elliott MJ, Caprise PA, Henning AE, Kurtz CA, Sekiya JK (2012) Diagnostic knee arthroscopy: a pilot study to evaluate surgical skills. Arthroscopy 28(2):218–224, available from: PM:22035780

Farnworth LR, Lemay DE, Wooldridge T, Mabrey JD, Blaschak MJ, DeCoster TA, Wascher DC, Schenck RC Jr (2001) A comparison of operative times in arthroscopic ACL reconstruction between orthopaedic faculty and residents: the financial impact of orthopaedic surgical training in the operating room. Iowa Orthop J 21:31–35, available from: PM:11813948

Guttmann D, Graham RD, MacLennan MJ, Lubowitz JH (2005) Arthroscopic rotator cuff repair: the learning curve. Arthroscopy 21(4):394–400, available from: PM:15800517

Harewood GC, Murray F, Winder S, Patchett S (2008) Evaluation of formal feedback on endoscopic competence among trainees: the EFFECT trial. Ir J Med Sci 177(3):253–256, available from: PM:18584274

Hodgins JL, Veillette C (2013) Arthroscopic proficiency: methods in evaluating competency. BMC Med Educ 13:61, available from: PM:23631421

Hoppe DJ, de Sa D, Simunovic N, Bhandari M, Safran MR, Larson CM, Ayeni OR (2014) The learning curve for hip arthroscopy: a systematic review. Arthroscopy, available from: PM:24461140

Howells NR, Gill HS, Carr AJ, Price AJ, Rees JL (2008) Transferring simulated arthroscopic skills to the operating theatre: a randomised blinded study. J Bone Joint Surg Br 90(4):494–499, available from: PM:18378926

Insel A, Carofino B, Leger R, Arciero R, Mazzocca AD (2009) The development of an objective model to assess arthroscopic performance. J Bone Joint Surg Am 91(9):2287–2295, available from: PM:19724008

Koehler RJ, Amsdell S, Arendt EA, Bisson LJ, Braman JP, Butler A, Cosgarea AJ, Harner CD, Garrett WE, Olson T, Warme WJ, Nicandri GT (2013) The arthroscopic surgical skill evaluation tool (ASSET). Am J Sports Med 41(6):1229–1237, available from: PM:23548808

Koehler RJ, Nicandri GT (2013) Using the arthroscopic surgery skill evaluation tool as a pass-fail examination. J Bone Joint Surg Am 95(23):e1871–e1876, available from: PM:24306710

Mabrey JD, Gillogly SD, Kasser JR, Sweeney HJ, Zarins B, Mevis H, Garrett WE Jr, Poss R, Cannon WD (2002) Virtual reality simulation of arthroscopy of the knee. Arthroscopy 18(6):E28, available from: PM:12098110

Martin JA, Regehr G, Reznick R, MacRae H, Murnaghan J, Hutchison C, Brown M (1997) Objective structured assessment of technical skill (OSATS) for surgical residents. Br J Surg 84(2):273–278, available from: PM:9052454

Matziolis G, Krocker D, Weiss U, Tohtz S, Perka C (2007) A prospective, randomized study of computer-assisted and conventional total knee arthroplasty. Three-dimensional evaluation of implant alignment and rotation. J Bone Joint Surg Am 89(2):236–243, available from: PM:17272435

Minekus JP, Rozing PM, Valstar ER, Dankelman J (2003) Evaluation of humeral head replacements using time-action analysis. J Shoulder Elbow Surg 12(2):152–157, available from: PM:12700568

Moon YW, Ha CW, Do KH, Kim CY, Han JH, Na SE, Lee CH, Kim JG, Park YS (2012) Comparison of robot-assisted and conventional total knee arthroplasty: a controlled cadaver study using multiparameter quantitative three-dimensional CT assessment of alignment. Comput Aided Surg 17(2):86–95, available from: PM:22348661

Morris AH, Jennings JE, Stone RG, Katz JA, Garroway RY, Hendler RC (1993) Guidelines for privileges in arthroscopic surgery. Arthroscopy 9(1):125–127, available from: PM:8442822

O'Connor A, Schwaitzberg SD, Cao CG (2008) How much feedback is necessary for learning to suture? Surg Endosc 22(7):1614–1619, available from: PM:17973165

O'Neill PJ, Cosgarea AJ, Freedman JA, Queale WS, McFarland EG (2002) Arthroscopic proficiency: a survey of orthopaedic sports medicine fellowship directors and orthopaedic surgery department chairs. Arthroscopy 18(7):795–800, available from: PM:12209439

Olson T, Koehler R, Butler A, Amsdell S, Nicandri G (2013) Is there a valid and reliable assessment of diagnostic knee arthroscopy skill? Clin Orthop Relat Res 471(5):1670–1676, available from: PM:23254692

Padoy N, Blum T, Ahmadi SA, Feussner H, Berger MO, Navab N (2012) Statistical modeling and recognition of surgical workflow. Med Image Anal 16(3):632–641, available from: PM:21195015

Pedowitz RA, Esch J, Snyder S (2002) Evaluation of a virtual reality simulator for arthroscopy skills development. Arthroscopy 18(6):E29, available from: PM:12098111

Prince M (2004) Does active learning work? A review of the research. J Eng Educ 93(3):223–231

Reznick R, Regehr G, MacRae H, Martin J, McCulloch W (1997) Testing technical skill via an innovative "bench station" examination. Am J Surg 173(3):226–230, available from: PM:9124632

Rosenberger RE, Hoser C, Quirbach S, Attal R, Hennerbichler A, Fink C (2008) Improved accuracy of component alignment with the implementation of image-free navigation in total knee arthroplasty. Knee Surg SportsTraumatol Arthrosc 16(3):249–257, available from: PM:18157493

Savoie FH III (2007) Guidelines to becoming an expert elbow arthroscopist. Arthroscopy 23(11):1237–1240, available from: PM:17986413

Sjoerdsma W, Meijer DW, Jansen A, den Boer KT, Grimbergen CA (2000) Comparison of efficiencies of three techniques for colon surgery. J Laparoendosc Adv Surg Tech A 10(1):47–53, available from: PM:10706303

Slade Shantz JA, Leiter JR, Collins JB, MacDonald PB (2013) Validation of a global assessment of arthroscopic skills in a cadaveric knee model. Arthroscopy 29(1):106–112, available from: PM:23177383

Tuijthof GJ, de Vaal MM, Sierevelt IN, Blankevoort L, van der List MP (2011) Performance of arthroscopic irrigation systems assessed with automatic blood detection. Knee Surg Sports Traumatol Arthrosc 19(11):1948–1954, available from: PM:21479643

Tuijthof GJ, Sierevelt IN, van Dijk CN (2007) Disturbances in the arthroscopic view defined with video analysis. Knee Surg Sports Traumatol Arthrosc 15(9):1101–1106, available from: PM:17410346

Tuijthof GJ, van den Boomen H, van Heerwaarden RJ, van Dijk CN (2008) Comparison of two arthroscopic pump systems based on image quality. Knee Surg Sports Traumatol Arthrosc 16(6):590–594, available from: PM:18322672

Van Oldenrijk J, Schafroth MU, Bhandari M, Runne WC, Poolman RW (2008) Time-action analysis (TAA) of the surgical technique implanting the collum femoris preserving (CFP) hip arthroplasty. TAASTIC trial identifying pitfalls during the learning curve of surgeons participating in a subsequent randomized controlled trial (an observational study). BMC Musculoskelet Disord 9:93, available from: PM:18577202

Guidelines and Concluding Remarks

14

Mustafa Karahan, Gino M.M.J. Kerkhoffs,
Pietro S. Randelli, and Gabriëlle J.M. Tuijthof

As stated in Chap. 1, an orthopaedic surgeon needs to be a *homo universalis* with obtaining arthroscopic skills being just one of the features that need to be trained into proficiency. In terms of technical skills, arthroscopic surgery has become the leading operative therapy for a growing number of injuries, due to its success in patient health care (Modi et al. 2010; Tuijthof et al. 2010). Since arthroscopy requires such a different manual handling compared to everyday life interactions with instruments (e.g. cutting paper with scissors or tightening a screw), it takes considerable time to become proficient. This implicates an increased risk of surgical errors during the early stages of the learning curve (Cannon et al. 2006; McCarthy et al. 2006; O'Neill et al. 2002).

In this education book, we have gathered the state-of-the-art knowledge, science, tools and equipment from relevant disciplines including education, neuroscience, mechanical and electrical engineering, computer science, endoscopy and evidence-based medicine that should provide educators the backbone to develop up-to-date training programmes that are effective and efficient and moreover keep the patients safe. Adequate basic training of arthroscopic skills is a must, as everybody knows that learning it the right way from scratch is the most effective manner. In addition to obtaining these basic skills, one should realise that surgeons need to keep them up to date and should be encouraged to do so in lifelong learning programmes. Thus, it is wise to make a plan that runs through the entire career of an orthopaedic surgeon. Advanced training of arthroscopic skills could, for example, imply advanced cadaver courses, fellowships, preparation of complex surgeries in patient-specific simulators and regular demonstration of competency.

To offer you an overall framework to start developing training programmes, we use the education theory of constructive alignment, which states that in a well-designed training programme three training elements are formulated explicitly and are aligned (Biggs 2003):

M. Karahan (✉)
Department of Orthopedics and Traumatology,
Acibadem University School of Medicine,
Istanbul, Turkey
e-mail: drmustafakarahan@gmail.com

GinoM.M.J.Kerkhoffs
Department of Orthopedic Surgery, Academic
Medical Centre, Amsterdam, The Netherlands
e-mail: g.m.kerkhoffs@amc.uva.nl

P.S. Randelli, MD
Aggregato in Ortopedia e Traumatologia,
Dipartimento Di Scienze Medico-Chirurgiche,
Ricercatore Università degli Studi di Milano, IRCCS
Policlinico San Donato, Milan, Italy
e-mail: pietro.randelli@unimi.it

G.J.M. Tuijthof
Department of Orthopedic Surgery, Academic
Medical Centre, Amsterdam, The Netherlands

Department of Biomechanical Engineering, Delft
University of Technology, Delft, The Netherlands

M. Karahan et al. (eds.), *Effective Training of Arthroscopic Skills*,
DOI 10.1007/978-3-662-44943-1_14, © ESSKA 2015

Learning objectives: What should be trained?

Means: How should it be trained?

Assessment: Is the objective achieved?

These three elements represent the three parts of the book and have been extensively elucidated. We will not repeat the take-home messages, but reflect upon each of the three training elements.

14.1 What Should Be Trained? What Are the Learning Objectives?

Chapters 2, 3 and 4 contributed to answering this question. Addressing the learning objectives can already be a difficult hurdle to take, not so much in defining the overall objective, which is training surgeons that are competent in applying, integrating and evaluating arthroscopic skills, medical knowledge and team skills. This is a precondition that contributes to safe, high-quality and efficient treatment. But formulating detailed learning objectives for each step in the overall training scheme can be challenging as experienced educators have automated their instrument handling such that it can be hard to describe what they do as they do not think about every step anymore (Chap. 3). Chapters 2, 3 and 4 provide you with a background theory, wishes from the arthroscopic community and practical suggestions to obtain and to maintain:

1. Basic arthroscopic skills (Chap. 2): Portal placement, anatomic knowledge on the identification of all important structures in the knee joint and inspection with the arthroscope
2. Automating arthroscopic skills (Chap. 3): Exposure to many different conditions and adoption of training conditions to innate characteristics of the trainee
3. Knowledge acquisition skills (Chap. 4): Integration of knowledge and skills and facilitating lifelong learning

A small addition to these chapters is that in defining learning objectives one can use the sequence of various surgical operation steps as described in operative protocols in combination with video analyses of arthroscopic procedures and seek agreement on the learning objectives with fellow educators *and* the trainees themselves.

14.2 How Should It Be Trained? What Are the Training Means?

Chapters 5, 6 and 7 gives a state-of-the-art overview of the ample availability of training means that can be used to implement in training programmes that ultimately lead to achieve the stated learning objectives. As discussed in Chaps. 8 and 9, each training means has its strong and limiting points. Not only the training means but aspects such as number of trainees, frequency, dexterity, performance measuring and feedback (Chap. 10) should be considered when developing a training module. Taking into account all these parameters – the learning objectives, validation evidence, costs, frequency of use, type of trainees, etc. – careful selection of the adequate training means is a difficult step. Once chosen, you can further detail and work out the training programme. Note that, supported by the theory on psychomotor learning, we claim that there is a place for all training means in a *perfect* lifelong training programme:

1. E-learning and arthroscopic videos offer a platform to learn arthroscopic anatomy, clinical variations and fundamentals of medical devices (Chaps. 2 and 4).
2. Dexterity tests highlight the innate capacities of a trainee and direct the pace and training content (Chap. 3 and 6).
3. Virtual reality simulators provide excellent conditions to train eye-hand coordination and technical procedural steps (Chap. 7).
4. Physical models allow additional training of safe tissue manipulation with actual instruments (Chap. 6).

5. Hands-on cadaver training is suitable for more advanced learners who wish to get acquainted with a new technique or device (Chap. 5).

All trainings means are no substitute for continued training in the operating room, but simply contribute highly to well-prepared and sufficiently competent residents, when continuing training in the operating room, and contribute to updating and maintaining the skills once proficiency has been achieved. The operating room offers the platform to train the integration of medical and equipment knowledge with psychomotor skills and team skills which lead to becoming the *homo universalis* (Chap. 4).

With the *perfect* training programme designed on paper, still quite some work has to be done to implement new training means into the curricula, as it takes time and money and in a number of cases additional scientific evidence to make the changes (Chaps. 8 and 9). We expect that governments and also institutes such as the ESSKA can play a crucial role by obligating the required changes, as is, for example, starting in the United Kingdom. Such initiatives will have a flywheel effect. Developers of training means will have their required market potential to further develop their products and offer them at reduced prices. Staff and faculty are encouraged to embrace new technology, increase the available content and above all prove that their training programmes are high quality and offer fair assessment. This will stimulate a set-up of the needed research in this area such as demonstrating the transfer validity of training means (Chap. 8), validating objective assessment criteria and high-quality training material and staff, and determining thresholds (Chap. 12) (Modi et al. 2010).

14.3   Is the Learning Objective Achieved? How Is It Assessed?

Chapters 11, 12 and 13 contributed to answering this question. Assessment is inextricably bound up with the learning objectives (Biggs 2003). For part tasks and basic skills, sufficient objective parameters are available that can be fairly easily implemented (e.g. the use of stopwatch), give insight to the training progress and allow comparison amongst peers (Chap. 11). The challenge is the actual implementation of those parameters in the current training programmes. We hope that this book has shown that to start measuring trainees activities can be as easy as to start using a stopwatch and will take away possible obstructions in logistics within the existing programmes. Another strong recommendation is to start implementing pre- and posttests in training programmes, which can give you valuable information on the quality of your course and determine if the trainees actually learn what you have planned.

Also, quite a few global rating scales (GRS) have recently been developed which can assess the overall skills in a more holistic approach (Chap. 13). Educators should be aware when using the GRS that observers should be trained properly and are in a position to give an objective judgment of the trainee's performance. This is especially important in summative judgment for which more developments need to be done. A final remark on assessment is to stimulate educators to define at least one parameter that can be measured both in a simulated environment and in the operating room, as this contributes to continued monitoring of training progress even in a lifelong training programme.

14.4   Conclusions

We hope to have inspired you to embrace new educational technologies and to start experimenting with implementing some of the work. For other enthusiasts, we hope to have stimulated you to continue innovative developments and perform necessary research in this area.

There is so much cool training equipment available and so much knowledge ready at hand that we feel it is merely a matter of time before all will be used. Not only because society demands that but also because our residents will request it. Do not forget that many of the new tools offer lots of fun in training as well. We are in this together so let us help each other, since we have a mutual goal of training the best surgeons now and in the future.

Bibliography

Biggs J (2003) Constructing learning by aligning teaching: constructive alignment. In: Biggs J (ed) Teaching for quality learning at university, 2nd edn. Open University Press, Berkshire, pp 11–33

Cannon WD, Eckhoff DG, Garrett WE Jr, Hunter RE, Sweeney HJ (2006) Report of a group developing a virtual reality simulator for arthroscopic surgery of the knee joint. Clin Orthop Relat Res 442:21–29, available from: PM:16394734

McCarthy AD, Moody L, Waterworth AR, Bickerstaff DR (2006) Passive haptics in a knee arthroscopy simulator: is it valid for core skills training? Clin Orthop Relat Res 442:13–20, available from: PM:16394733

Modi CS, Morris G, Mukherjee R (2010) Computer-simulation training for knee and shoulder arthroscopic surgery. Arthroscopy 26(6):832–840, available from: PM:20511043

O'Neill PJ, Cosgarea AJ, Freedman JA, Queale WS, McFarland EG (2002) Arthroscopic proficiency: a survey of orthopaedic sports medicine fellowship directors and orthopaedic surgery department chairs. Arthroscopy 18(7):795–800, available from: PM:12209439

Tuijthof GJ, van Sterkenburg MN, Sierevelt IN, Van OJ, van Dijk CN, Kerkhoffs GM (2010) First validation of the PASSPORT training environment for arthroscopic skills. Knee Surg Sports Traumatol Arthrosc 18(2):218–224, available from: PM:19629441

Index